NUCLEAR REGULATORY COMMISSION REGULATION OF NUCLEAR MEDICINE

Guide for Diagnostic Nuclear Medicine and Radiopharmaceutical Therapy

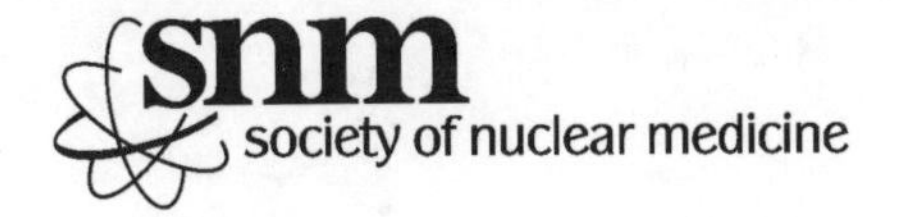

Society of Nuclear Medicine, Inc.
1850 Samuel Morse Drive
Reston, VA 20190-5316

Made in the United States of America.

Library of Congress Cataloging-in-Publication Data

Guide for diagnostic nuclear medicine and radiopharmaceutical therapy / [edited by] Jeffry A. Siegel.
p. ; cm.
Includes bibliographical references and index.
ISBN 0-9726478-2-1
1. Radioisotope scanning. 2. Nuclear medicine. 3. Radiopharmaceuticals. 4. Radioisotopes in pharmacology.
[DNLM: 1. Nuclear Medicine--organization & administration--United States--Legislation. 2. Nuclear Medicine--standards--United States--Legislation. 3. Diagnostic Techniques, Radioisotope--standards--United States--Legislation. 4. Radiation Monitoring--standards--United States--Legislation. 5. Radiation Protection--standards--United States--Legislation. 6. Radiotherapy--standards--United States--Legislation. WN 440 G946 2004] I. Siegel, Jeffry A. II. Society of Nuclear Medicine (1953-)
RC78.7.R4G85 2004
616.07'575--dc22

2004010618
2004010652

Contents

Guide for Radiopharmaceutical Therapy

Foreword

In a 1954 staff memorandum submitted to the Atomic Energy Commission (AEC), it was proposed that general radiological health and safety standards be added to the AEC regulations. Minimal requirements were set forth, but no attempt was made to specify the exact means of compliance. It was specifically stated that, "The methods or procedures to be used in complying with the regulations are left to the discretion of the user inasmuch as several optional procedures, equally efficacious, may be available in any particular case to assure minimum radiation exposure." The AEC thus decided 50 years ago that the safety standards provided in the regulations were sufficient and that there was no need to codify methods or procedures to be used in complying with the regulations. This does not necessarily imply that the AEC took the position that providing guidance to licensees was unnecessary; it may have been the product of the early state of development of regulatory oversight for peaceful uses of nuclear energy.

In today's regulatory environment, the Nuclear Regulatory Commission (NRC) believes that providing guidance to licensees for complying with its regulations is necessary and has developed many guidance documents over the years. When NRC recently revised 10 CFR Part 35, "Medical Use of Byproduct Material," effective on October 24, 2002, it also provided licensing guidance in NUREG-1556, Volume 9, "Consolidated Guidance About Materials Licenses, Program-Specific Guidance About Medical License," issued in October 2002. All diagnostic nuclear medicine and radiopharmaceutical therapy facilities must reevaluate their procedures and protection programs to determine whether they remain in compliance and what, if any, remedial actions are necessary. At the same time, the NRC's new risk-informed, performance-based approach focuses not on procedures but on outcomes. Specific courses of action are not prescribed, and operating policies and procedures may vary widely with modality, specific application, and size and type of institution.

There is no question that licensees must comply with NRC regulations, but doing so by adopting regulatory guidance is not necessary. NRC has clearly stated that its guidance for licensing under 10 CFR Part 35 is not intended to be the only means of satisfying requirements for a license. NRC guidance documents applicable to diagnostic nuclear medicine and radiopharmaceutical therapy represent only one means by which a licensee can comply with the regulations, and licensees are free to propose other methods.

The Joint Government Relations Committee of the American College of Nuclear Physicians (ACNP) and the Society of Nuclear Medicine (SNM) recognized that practitioners across the spectrum of diagnostic nuclear medicine and radiopharmaceutical therapy would value professional guidance in meeting the new outcomes requirements. This book is intended to serve as a useful bridge between the new regulations and practitioners who want to ensure continued compliance and maintain the security and safety of licensed materials in clinical and research settings. Unlike NUREG-1556, Volume 9, which provides licensing guidance for *all* medical uses of byproduct material, the SNM/ACNP Guide is limited to providing guidance to diagnostic nuclear medicine and radiopharmaceutical therapy practitioners. Working closely with representatives from the NRC, we developed a complete "walk-through" of the applicable regulations, focusing on the radiation protection program and implementation procedures necessary for compliance. We have also attempted to point out procedures that may not be necessary or that may be necessary to establish the documented radiation safety track record necessary for a licensee to unilaterally revise its radiation protection program to discontinue or modify certain components. "At a Glance" boxes throughout the book summarize the most important regulatory issues and pertinent regulations.

This book may be used by diagnostic nuclear medicine and radiopharmaceutical therapy practitioners in place of NUREG-1556, Volume 9. The NRC views this SNM/ACNP Guide "as providing focused information that may be useful to nuclear medicine professionals in understanding the applicability of NRC requirements to the medical use of byproduct material in diagnostic and radiopharmaceutical therapy settings, and as providing measures that practitioners in these settings may use to facilitate implementation of the revised rule."

We have differed from the standard NRC style in this volume in two minor ways. First, because the book is intended as a ready reference, we have spelled out all abbreviations the first time (and only the first time) they appear in each chapter and in each of the very lengthy main subheadings of Chapters 9 and 16. A list of abbreviations is included on page xii. Second, we have provided all measures of radiation and/or radioactivity as conventional units followed in parentheses by the equivalent measure expressed in Système Internationale units.

We have worked to ensure that all information in this book is accurate as of the time of publication and consistent with standards of good practice. As research and practice advance, however, standards may change. For this reason it is recommended that readers evaluate the applicability of any recommendations in light of specific situations and changing standards. In addition, because this book recommends licensing guidance compatible with NRC regulations, not all recommendations will apply in Agreement States.

This volume represents the first attempt by a stakeholder professional organization to give alternate and stand-alone guidance and, in agreement with the 1954 AEC staff position, the model procedures are merely samples and not minimum standards. For all practitioners, the primary and paramount focus remains on the accurate, timely, and safe diagnosis and treatment of illness and disease. Compliance with changing federal regulations and increased familiarity with the implications of these regulations will assure both practitioners and patients of adequate and effective radiation safety practices.

Jeffry A. Siegel, PhD
Chair, Joint Government Relations Committee
American College of Nuclear Physicians/Society of Nuclear Medicine

Acknowledgments

This work was a collaborative effort by volunteer professionals in the nuclear medicine sciences in cooperation with the staffs of the Society of Nuclear Medicine (SNM) and the Nuclear Regulatory Commission (NRC). Alan H. Maurer, MD, was among those who first proposed the need for such a volume, and it was through his organizational efforts that work on the project began. The draft was reviewed by the SNM Board of Directors, the American College of Nuclear Physicians (ACNP) Board of Regents, the Members of the ACNP/SNM Government Relations Committee, and members and staff of the American College of Radiology, the American Society for Therapeutic Radiology and Oncology and the American College of Medical Physics. NRC staff provided additional information. Of special assistance in the process of identifying topics to be covered, facilitating preparation and publication, and maintaining productive liaisons with the NRC were Virginia Pappas, CAE, SNM Executive Director, William Uffelman, JD, SNM General Counsel and Director of Public Affairs, and G. Rebecca Haines, SNM Director of Publications.

Peer reviewers for the draft included:

Robert Forrest
Radiation Safety Officer
University of Pennsylvania
Philadelphia, PA

John P. Jacobus, MS, CHP
Health Physicist
National Institutes of Health
Bethesda, MD

Alan H. Maurer, MD
Temple University Hospital
Philadelphia, PA

Peter G. Vernig
Radiation Safety Officer
VA Medical Center
Denver, CO

Revision reviewers for the draft included:

Sue H. Abreu, MD
Robert W. Atcher, PhD
Jorge R. Barrio, PhD
Terence Beven, MD
Manuel L. Brown, MD
Roy Brown
Mickey T. Clarke, CNMT
R. Edward Coleman, MD
Peter S. Conti, MD
Valerie R. Cronin, CNMT
Simindokt Dadparvar, MD
Gary Dillehay, MD
Lynne A. Fairobent
Lynnette A. Fulk, CNMT
Michael J. Gelfand, MD
Leonie L. Gordon, MD
Bennett S. Greenspan, MD
Robert E. Henkin, MD
Frances K. Keech, RT(N), MBA
Peter T. Kirchner, MD
Steven M. Larson, MD
Letty G. Lutzker, MD
Kenneth A. McKusick, MD
Carol Marcus, MD
Lyn M. Mehlberg
Denise A. Merlino, MBA
Warren H. Moore, MD
Paul H. Murphy, PhD
Virginia Pappas, CAE
Patrick J. Peller, MD
Thomas R. Pounds, MD
Lynne T. Roy, CNMT
Henry D. Royal, MD
Edward M. Smith, ScD
Daniel E. Stobbe, MD
Mathew L. Thakur, PhD
LisaAnn Trembath, BA, CNMT
Mark Tulchinsky, MD
Harish Vaidya, CNMT, NCT
William A. Van Decker, MD
Doug Van Nostrand, MD
Robert H. Wagner, MD
Hadyn T. Williams, MD
Michael A. Wilson, MD
Randall S. Winn, MD
Louis S. Zeiger, MD

Abbreviations

AEA	Atomic Energy Act
AEC	Atomic Energy Commission
ALARA	as low as reasonably achievable
ALI	annual limit on intake
AMP	authorized medical physicist
ANP	authorized nuclear pharmacist
AU	authorized user
CDE	committed dose equivalent
CEDE	committed effective dose equivalent
cft	cubic feet
CRCPD	Conference of Radiation Control Program Directors
DAC	derived air concentration
DCF	dose conversion factor
DDE	deep-dose equivalent
DOE	U.S. Department of Energy
EDE	effective dose equivalent
FDA	U.S. Food and Drug Administration
IND	Investigational New Drug
LDE	lens dose equivalent
LNT	linear nonthreshold model
NCRP	National Council on Radiation Protection and Measurements
NRC	U.S. Nuclear Regulatory Commission (here, also, the Commission)
NVLAP	National Voluntary Laboratory Accreditation Program
OSL	optically stimulated luminescent dosimeter
RDRC	Radioactive Drug Research Committee
RSO	radiation safety officer
SDE	shallow-dose equivalent
TEDE	total effective dose equivalent
TLD	thermoluminescent dosimeter
TODE	total organ dose equivalent

Guide for
Diagnostic Nuclear Medicine

1 Introduction

1.1 Background

This section of the book was developed to provide guidance to diagnostic nuclear medicine applicants and/or licensees in the implementation of the U.S. Nuclear Regulatory Commission's (NRC's) newly revised 10 CFR Part 35, *Medical Use of Byproduct Material.* This guidance is aimed at all diagnostic nuclear medicine licensees using unsealed byproduct material for uptake, dilution, excretion, and imaging and localization studies for which a written directive (i.e., a written order for the administration of byproduct material to a specific patient or human research subject) is not required. The regulations require that applicants and/or licensees develop, document, and implement operating policies and procedures as part of an overall radiation protection program that will ensure compliance and the security and safe use of licensed materials. These radiation protection policies and implementing procedures are neither detailed in the regulations nor required to be submitted as part of the license application.

Some diagnostic nuclear medicine practitioners have developed their own radiation protection programs, but most have relied on model procedures published by the NRC in guidance documents. NUREG-1556, Volume 9, *Consolidated Guidance About Material Licenses: Program-Specific Guidance About Medical Use Licenses,* provides guidance on the revised Part 35 rule. Adoption of the NRC licensing guidance is not mandatory. Information in NUREG-1556, Volume 9, describes one acceptable method to comply with 10 CFR Part 35. Licensees may propose other methods. However, in all cases licensees are responsible for compliance with Part 35.

1.2 Need for This Report

Currently, NRC requirements and licensing guidance for diagnostic and therapeutic medicine are intermingled. This section of this book represents the first attempt by a stakeholder professional organization, in this case the Society of Nuclear Medicine and the American College of Nuclear Physicians, to develop a separate document applicable to the practice of diagnostic nuclear medicine. The suggested operating policies and procedures are the minimum necessary to ensure compliance with the revised Part 35 regulations and with other NRC regulations (e.g., certain requirements contained in 10 CFR Parts 19, 20, and 30) that are applicable to diagnostic nuclear medicine licensees. *It must be emphasized that the model procedures in this book are merely samples and must not be considered minimum standards.*

The NRC has adopted a risk-informed, performance-based approach to regulation. The result is that the procedural aspects of a licensee's radiation protection program are not required to constitute "best practice" in the medical use of radionuclides, as long as performance outcomes are in compliance. The continued need for some of the suggested procedures in this book should be considered in light of the licensee's own prior experience obtained during reviews of its radiation protection program. It may be prudent for new applicants/licensees to implement the procedures as written, whereas established licensees should revise and/or essentially eliminate unnecessary procedures. For example, if a licensee, after continual review of worker dose histories, determines that no individual has received a radiation dose in excess of the applicable limits, monitoring of workers could potentially be eliminated. However, vigilance should be maintained to ensure that current programs continue to meet regulatory requirements.

1.3 Scope and Application

The radiation protection policies and implementing procedures suggested in this section were developed based on NRC regulations. They may not apply to diagnostic nuclear medicine facilities in Agreement States. It will be necessary, therefore, even for those wishing to adopt a template procedure in Agreement States, to review procedures against the medical use regulations and other requirements of their state.

Because the NRC also has committed to a risk-informed, performance-based approach to inspection, guidance documents such as the suggested operating policies and procedures in this book should not be used as the primary inspection criteria, except in the event of a performance failure. It must be considered that procedural omissions or lapses in teaching or supervision of nuclear medicine technologists in these procedures are not the reasons for every misstep.

Readers will have here, for the first time in one place, all the NRC regulations and radiation protection policies and implementing procedures applicable to diagnostic nuclear medicine. Therapeutic procedures that require a written directive are covered in the second section of this book. It is hoped that all nuclear medicine practitioners will read these requirements and suggested operating policies and procedures necessary for compliance. This should serve not only as a valuable educational tool but also as a resource for all diagnostic nuclear medicine and radiopharmaceutical therapy professionals. It is our hope that both sections of this book will be used both in the license application process and in the development and continual evaluation of individual licensee risk-informed, performance-based radiation protection programs.

2

The Practice of Diagnostic Nuclear Medicine

2.1 Diagnostic Nuclear Medicine

Diagnostic nuclear medicine began more than 50 years ago and has evolved into a major medical specialty. Its practitioners use low activity levels of radioactive materials in a safe way to gain information about health and disease. Small amounts of radioactive materials, known as radiopharmaceuticals, are introduced into the body by injection, swallowing, or inhalation. Different radiopharmaceuticals are used to study different parts of the body. These agents emit photons that can be detected externally by special cameras. These cameras produce images on film and/or work in conjunction with computers to produce images of the body's organs. An estimated 12–14 million nuclear medicine procedures are performed each year in the United States. Diagnostic nuclear medicine studies determine the cause of a medical problem based on organ function, in contrast to radiographic studies, which determine the presence of disease based on structural appearance.

2.2 Diagnostic Nuclear Medicine Facility

A typical nuclear medicine facility contains the following rooms or areas:

(1) Reception area;
(2) File room;
(3) Waiting room;
(4) Hot lab;
(5) Imaging room(s);
(6) Thyroid uptake room;
(7) Physician office(s);
(8) Chief technologist office;
(9) Hallways; and
(10) Bathroom(s).

For regulatory purposes these areas are considered to be either restricted or unrestricted. Restricted areas are those to which access is limited by the licensee for the purpose of protecting individuals against unnecessary risks from exposure to radiation and radioactive materials. Usually, the hot lab, imaging room(s), and thyroid uptake room are considered restricted areas. Unrestricted areas are those areas to which access is neither limited nor controlled by the licensee.

Many devices and materials are used by diagnostic nuclear medicine licensees to ensure the safe use of radioactive materials and demonstrate compliance with applicable NRC regulations. In most facilities, these include but are not limited to:

(1) Dose calibrator;
(2) Fume hood;
(3) Shielding material (such as lead and leaded glass for use in the hot lab, pigs, syringe holders, syringe shields, aprons, and portable shields);
(4) Protective clothing (laboratory coats and gloves);
(5) Radioactive waste storage containers;
(6) Sealed calibration sources (for dose calibrator, well counter, and gamma camera);
(7) Survey meters and exposure meters;
(8) Well counter;
(9) Whole-body/ring dosimeters; and
(10) Individual room exhaust systems and activated charcoal gas traps.

2.3 Safety of Nuclear Medicine

Since the first use of nuclear medicine in the United States, more than one-third of a billion doses have been administered to patients, with a track record for safety that is unparalleled. The radiation dose associated with diagnostic nuclear medicine procedures averages 440 mrem (4.4 mSv) effective dose equivalent, according to a National Council on Radiation Protection and

Measurements study published in 1991. This average dose is even lower today as a result of increased use of radiopharmaceuticals labeled with ^{99m}Tc. Individuals living in most areas of the United States receive a comparable annual average dose (300 mrem [3 mSv]) from natural background radiation.

2.4 Radionuclides

The following radionuclides are most commonly used in diagnostic nuclear medicine procedures: ^{99m}Tc, ^{201}Tl, ^{67}Ga, ^{111}In, ^{123}I, ^{131}I, ^{133}Xe, and ^{18}F. All except ^{99m}Tc, ^{131}I, and ^{133}Xe are produced in particle accelerators and are not under the control of the NRC (but may be regulated by the states; see Chapter 5). The various positron-emitting radiopharmaceuticals used in positron emission tomography are also produced by particle accelerators. Radiation doses received from common diagnostic nuclear medicine procedures using these radionuclides and their typical administered activities are shown in Table 2.1.

Because of the low administered activities and short half-lives of these and other radiopharmaceuticals in the practice of diagnostic nuclear medicine, the resulting radiation doses (both organ doses in rad and effective dose equivalents in rem) pose extremely low radiation risks.

2.4.1 Radionuclides in Pregnancy and Breast Feeding

If a pregnant patient undergoes a diagnostic nuclear medicine procedure, the embryo/fetus will be exposed to radiation. Typical embryo/fetus radiation doses for more than 80 radiopharmaceuticals have been determined by Russell et al. (*Health Phys.* 1997;73: 756–769). For the most common diagnostic procedures in nuclear medicine, the doses range from 0.5×10^{-4} to 3.8 rad, the highest doses being for ^{67}Ga. Most procedures result in a dose that is a factor of 10 or more lower than the 3.8 rad dose.

In situations involving the administration of radiopharmaceuticals to women who are lactating, the breast feeding infant or child will be exposed to radiation through intake of radioactivity in the milk, as well as external exposure from close proximity to the mother. Radiation doses from the activity ingested by the infant have been estimated for the most common radiopharmaceuticals used in diagnostic nuclear medicine by Stabin and Breitz (*J Nucl Med.* 2000;41:862–873). In most cases, no interruption in breast feeding was needed to maintain a radiation dose to the infant well below 100 mrem (1 mSv). Only brief interruption (hours to days) of breast feeding was advised for ^{99m}Tc-macroaggregated albumin, ^{99m}Tc-pertechnetate, ^{99m}Tc-red blood cells, ^{99m}Tc-white blood cells, ^{123}I-metaiodobenzylguanidine, and ^{201}Tl. Complete cessation was suggested for ^{67}Ga-citrate, ^{123}I-sodium iodide, and ^{131}I-sodium iodide. The recommendation for ^{123}I was based on a 2.5% contamination with ^{125}I, which is no longer applicable.

2.5 Radiation Effects and Risk Estimates

Concerns about stochastic radiogenic risks have led to NRC regulations for diagnostic nuclear medicine that inherently demand a radiation protection philosophy based on the conservative hypothesis that some risk is associated with even the smallest doses of radiation. There is no question that exposure of any individual to potential risk, however low, should be minimized if it can be readily avoided or is not accompanied by some benefit. The weighing of risks and benefits, however, is not always based on objective data and calls for personal value judgments, which can vary widely.

In 1901, 5 years after discovering radioactivity, Henri Becquerel recognized the risks involved in exposure to radioactive isotopes. A short time after he had carried a sample of uranium in his pocket, he observed that the underlying skin developed first erythema and then tissue necrosis, which he attributed to the radioactive properties of the specimen. Today, after more than a century of careful review of the evidence for radiation effects from the radiation doses associated with diagnostic nuclear medicine, there appears to be little reason for apprehension about either genetic or somatic effects (including thyroid cancer).

2.5.1 Deterministic and Stochastic Effects

The biologic effects of ionizing radiation are divided into two classes: deterministic and stochastic.

A deterministic effect occurs every time a certain radiation dose level (or threshold dose) is exceeded. Deterministic effects include reddening of the skin, sterility, cataracts, radiation sickness, and even death if the

TABLE 2.1

Radiation Doses from Common Diagnostic Nuclear Medicine Procedures*

Radionuclide	Agent	Typical administered** activities (mCi)	Highest dose (organ)** (rad)	EDE (rem)
^{18}F	FDG	10	5.9 (bladder)	0.7
^{67}Ga	Citrate	5	11.8 (bone surfaces)	1.9
^{99m}Tc	HIDA	5	2.0 (gallbladder)	0.3
	HMPAO	20	2.5 (kidneys)	0.7
	MAA	4	1.0 (lungs)	0.2
	MDP	20	4.7 (bone surfaces)	0.4
	MAG3 (normal function)	20	8.1 (bladder wall)	0.5
	DTPA	10	2.3 (bladder wall)	0.2
	Sestamibi			
	Rest	20	2.9 (gallbladder)	0.7
	Stress	20	2.4 (gallbladder)	0.6
	Sulfur colloid	8	2.2 (spleen)	0.3
	Tetrofosmin			
	Rest	20	2.7 (gallbladder)	0.6
	Stress	20	2.0 (gallbladder)	0.5
^{111}In	White blood cells	0.5	10.9 (spleen)	1.2
^{123}I	NaI (25% uptake)	0.4	2.8 (thyroid)	0.2
	MIBG	0.4	0.1 (liver)	0.02
^{131}I	NaI (25% uptake)	0.02	26.6 (thyroid)	0.8
	MIBG	0.02	0.06 (liver)	0.01
^{133}Xe	Gas	15	0.06 (lungs)	0.04
^{201}Tl	Chloride	2	4.6 (thyroid)	1.2

* Adapted from Bushberg JT, Seibert JA, Leidholdt EM, Boone JM. *The Essential Physics of Medical Imaging.* 2d ed. Philadelphia, PA: Lippincott Williams & Wilkins; in press; 2002; available on-line at www.doseinfo-radar.com.)

** SI conversion: 1 rem = 0.01 Sv; 1 mCi = 37 MBq.

EDE = effective dose equivalent; FDG = fluorodeoxyglucose; HIDA = hepatic iminodiacetic acid; HMPAO = hexamethylpropyleneamine oxime; MAA = macroaggregated albumin; MDP = methylene diphosphonate; MAG3 = mercaptoacetyltriglycine; DTPA = diethylenetriaminepentaacetic acid; MIBG = metaiodobenzylguanidine.

dose is high enough. Deterministic effects occur only after relatively high dose levels that exceed the threshold for those effects, usually a dose on the order of 100 rem (1 Sv). Therefore, the risk of deterministic effects attributed to the exposures likely to be encountered in diagnostic nuclear medicine procedures is insignificant.

Stochastic effects happen only to a certain percentage of individuals in a group that is exposed to a given hazard. A good example of a stochastic effect is cancer caused by cigarette smoking. Not everyone who smokes heavily will get cancer, but their chances of getting cancer are increased by smoking heavily. The principal stochastic effect from radiation doses associated with diagnostic nuclear medicine is cancer. Hereditary effects manifested in the offspring of exposed individuals are less likely. In a large population exposed to a low dose of radiation, only a few of the individuals will be affected. Some cancers are more likely to occur than others, and the time for them to develop (the latent period) varies. The risk of stochastic effects increases as a function of radiation dose.

(For deterministic effects, the severity increases as a function of dose, but only after a threshold dose has been exceeded.)

To determine the risk of stochastic effects associated with low doses of radiation, a model is typically applied using the observed effects in individuals exposed to high doses of radiation delivered over a short period of time (e.g., studies of survivors of the atomic bomb). These data are extrapolated down to "estimated" effects at low radiation doses and dose rates. The dose–effect relationships are estimates based on the linear nonthreshold (LNT) model. There have been no observed effects at the low doses encountered in daily life as a result of radiation exposure from, for example, background radiation, consumer products, or diagnostic nuclear medicine. Considering that the normal incidence of cancer in the population of the United States is approximately 40%, even the most conservative cancer risk estimates at the low doses inherent to diagnostic nuclear medicine are extremely low and probably would not be detectable.

2.5.2 The Linear Nonthreshold Model

The current (conservative) public health practice is to base low-dose risk estimates on the LNT model. A position statement by the Health Physics Society in 1996 (Mossman KL. *Health Phys.* 1996;70:749–750), however, recommended against quantitative estimation of health risk below an individual dose of 5 rem (0.05 Sv) in 1 year, which is the occupational dose limit for adult radiation workers. At these levels, noted the statement, the risks of health effects are either too small to be observed or are nonexistent. A recent review of health hazards after exposures to background radiation, radon in homes, medical procedures, and occupational radiation in large population samples by investigators at the National Institutes of Health (Ernst M, Freed ME, Zametkin AJ. *J Nucl Med.* 1998;39:689–698) could not detect any health risks from low-level radiation above the "noise" of adverse events of everyday life. Having said that, the NRC requires that each licensee not only achieve doses to workers and to the public that are within regulatory limits but also maintain these doses as low as reasonably achievable.

3

History and Organization of Regulation of Nuclear Medicine

3.1 Brief History

The medical importance of radioisotopes was recognized before World War II, but distribution was unregulated by the government. In 1942, the Manhattan Project was begun by the United States Army to conduct atomic research with the goal of ending World War II. The postwar program for distributing radioisotopes grew out of the part of the Manhattan Project that had developed the greatest technical expertise with radionuclides during the war, the Isotopes Division at Oak Ridge, TN. In 1946, the Manhattan Project publicly announced its program for distributing radioactive isotopes for research purposes. Radioisotopes for medical research use could not simply be ordered; each purchase had to be reviewed and approved. For human applications, each application was reviewed by a special subcommittee.

The authority to continue this radioisotope research was transferred from the Army to the United States Atomic Energy Commission (AEC) by congressional passage of the Atomic Energy Act (AEA) of 1946. This act was signed into law by President Truman and gave the AEC a government monopoly in the field of atomic research and development. President Truman appointed David Lilienthal, former head of the Tennessee Valley Authority, as the first chair of the AEC. The review subcommittee for the AEC was renamed the Subcommittee on Human Applications, and, on June 28, 1946, this subcommittee held its first meeting. The members were Dr. Andrew Dowdy, chair, biophysicist Gioacchino Failla, and Dr. Hymer Friedell, executive officer of the Manhattan Project's Medical Section (who was not in attendance). Attending as nonvoting secretary was Paul Aebersold, in charge of the production of radioisotopes at Oak Ridge (later to head the AEC's Isotopes Division), and advisers W.E. Cohn and Karl Z. Morgan, director of Health Physics at Oak Ridge.

During this meeting, a system of local committees was suggested. Each local committee (or "local isotope committee") would include: (1) a physician well versed in the physiology and pathology of the blood forming organs; (2) a physician well versed in metabolism and metabolic disorders; and (3) a competent biophysicist, radiologist, or radiation physiologist qualified in the techniques of radioisotopes. By October 1946, the distribution program was well under way, with 217 requests received. Of these, 211 had been approved. Human use requests totaled 94, of which 90 had been approved. In 1959, the Subcommittee on Human Applications was absorbed into the Advisory Committee on Medical Uses of Isotopes.

Even as it developed procedures for unusual cases, the subcommittee recognized that some existing uses were becoming routine and did not need to be reviewed continuously by the subcommittee. The subcommittee delegated the review of such requests to the Isotopes Division. The Isotopes Division of the AEC developed a procedure whereby a person desiring to procure byproduct materials had to file an application and receive an Authorization for Radioisotope Procurement before obtaining and using byproduct materials. The authorization functioned in much the same way as a license. An additional simplification came with the introduction in 1951 of "General Authorizations," which delegated more authority to the local radioisotope committees of approved institutions. These authorizations enabled research institutions to obtain certain radioisotopes for approved purposes after filing a single application each year, thereby eliminating the need to file a separate application for each radioisotope order.

Throughout the 1950s, changes in the regulations affected administrative procedures. The AEA of 1954 added licensing and regulation to the authority of the AEC. Other concerns about radioisotope use were disseminated through circulars, brochures, and guides by the Isotopes Division. From the early 1960s until the early 1970s, the AEC was chaired by Glenn Seaborg, a Nobel laureate chemist who had been associated with the Metallurgical Laboratory in Chicago during World War II. The AEC was led subsequently by an economist and finally by a marine biologist (Dr. Dixy Lee Ray, the first woman to chair the AEC). In 1975, the AEC was split into the Energy Research and Development Administration (later to become the Department of Energy) and the Nuclear Regulatory Commission (NRC), as a result of congressional passage of the Energy Reorganization Act of 1974.

In 1948, the official circular describing medical applications was only three pages long. By 1957, it had been replaced by a 26-page guide, *The Medical Uses of Radioisotopes—Recommendations and Requirements* by the AEC. In 1965, the AEC published the *Guide for the Preparation of Applications for the Medical Use of Radioisotopes,* and, in 1980, the NRC published Regulatory Guide 10.8, *Guide for the Preparation of Applications for Medical Programs.* Many changes to NRC regulations and licensing guidance have occurred since this guide, including major revisions to 10 CFR Parts 20 and 35 and the publication of NUREG-1556, Volume 9, *Consolidated Guidance About Material Licenses: Program-Specific Guidance About Medical Use Licenses,* which provides guidance on the revised Part 35 rule.

3.2 Nuclear Regulatory Commission Organizational Overview

The 2002 NRC organizational overview (abbreviated) for the regulation of the medical use of byproduct material is shown in Figure 3.1. Additional information about the organizational structure of the NRC is available at www.nrc.gov.

FIGURE 3.1
Organization of the Nuclear Regulatory Commission

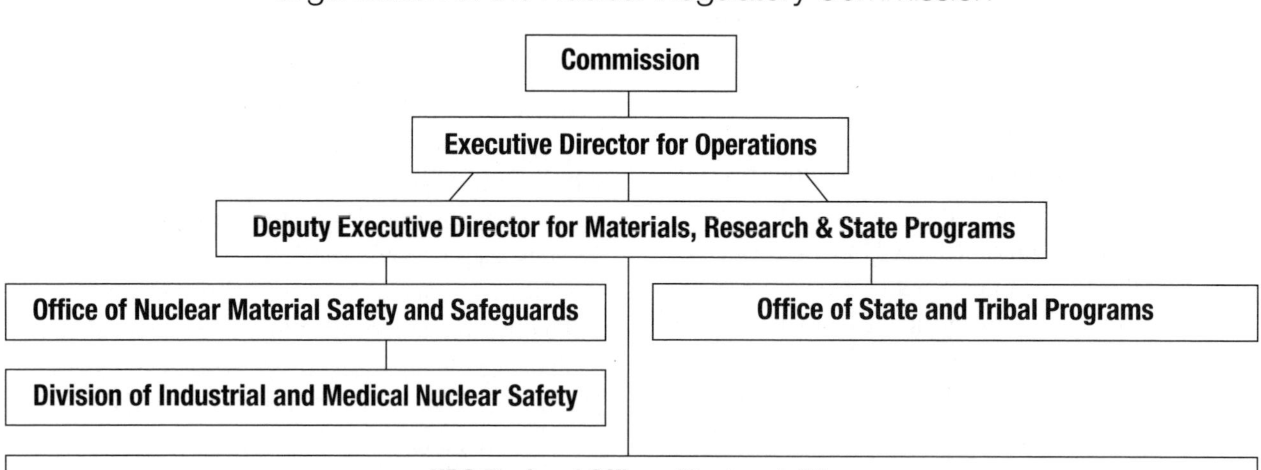

NRC Regional Offices (Regions I–IV)			
Region I	**Region II**	**Region III**	**Region IV**
Connecticut, Delaware, District of Columbia, New Hampshire, New Jersey, New York, Maine, Maryland, Massachusetts, Rhode Island, Vermont 475 Allendale Road King of Prussia, PA 19406-1415 800-432-1156	Alabama, Florida, Georgia, Kentucky, Mississippi, Puerto Rico, North Carolina, South Carolina, Tennessee, Virgin Islands, Virginia, West Virginia Atlanta Federal Center 61 Forsyth Street, SW, Suite 23T85 Atlanta, GA 30303-3415 800-577-8510	Illinois, Indiana, Iowa, Michigan, Minnesota, Missouri, Ohio, Wisconsin 801 Warrenville Road Lisle, IL 60532-4351 800-522-3025	Arizona, Arkansas, California, Colorado, Idaho, Kansas, Louisiana, Montana, Nebraska, Nevada, New Mexico, North Dakota, Oklahoma, Oregon, South Dakota, Texas, Utah, Washington, Wyoming 611 Ryan Plaza Drive, Suite 400 Arlington, TX 76011-8064 800-952-9677

4

Overview of Nuclear Regulatory Commission Regulations Applicable to Medical Use Licensees

4.1 Background

In the past, the Nuclear Regulatory Commission (NRC) accomplished its mission through regulation and license conditions. Because the NRC is shifting to a risk-informed, performance-based environment, certain license conditions may no longer be necessary. Historic precedents support this latter change of practice. For example, in a 1954 memorandum, S.R. Sapirie, manager of Oak Ridge Operations, stated that any radiological safety standard adopted by the then Atomic Energy Commission (AEC) should be published in the *Federal Register,* the designated central repository for all federal regulations. The memorandum also stated that "no person shall in any manner be required to resort to organizations or procedure not so published" (http://search.dis.anl.gov/plweb-cgi/mhrexpage.pl?0726743+1+27+_free). In 1966, AEC Chair Glenn Seaborg appointed a Radioisotopes Licensing Review Panel to review the regulations of the Commission. One of the conclusions of the panel was that emphasis on the licensee's own responsibilities for developing safe radiation practices would produce better results than detailed regulation and licensing conditions (http://search.dis.anl.gov/plweb-cgi/mhrexpage.pl?0717604+1+65+_free).

The NRC is bound by statute to regulate byproduct material as well as source and special nuclear material "to protect health and minimize danger to life or property." Section 161 of the Atomic Energy Act of 1954, as amended, authorized the AEC to establish by rule, regulation, or order "such standards and instructions to govern the possession and use of these materials as the Commission may deem necessary or desirable and to prescribe such regulations or orders as it may deem necessary to govern an activity authorized pursuant to the Act in order to protect health and/or minimize danger to life or property." NRC regulations governing the medical use of byproduct material are codified in Title 10 of the Code of Federal Regulations and are published in the *Federal Register.* The *Federal Register* is published by the Office of the Federal Register, National Archives and Records Administration, and is the official daily publication for rules, proposed rules, and notices of federal agencies and organizations, as well as executive orders and other presidential documents.

4.2 Title 10 CFR Parts Applicable to Medical Use Licensees

The following Parts of Title 10 CFR contain NRC regulations applicable to medical use licensees: Parts 2, 19, 20, 21, 30, 31, 32, 33, 35, 40, 70, 71, 150, 170, and 171. The Department of Energy and its prime contractors are exempt from NRC licensing (10 CFR 30.12). The major Parts of Title 10 that are applicable to diagnostic nuclear medicine licensees are Parts 19, 20, 30, and 35.

Part 19 Notices, Instructions, and Reports to Workers: Inspection and Investigations.
Contains requirements for posting of notices to workers, instructions to workers, reports of radiation exposure, and options available to workers for NRC inspections regarding radiological working conditions.

Part 20 Standards for Protection Against Radiation.
Contains general radiation protection requirements applicable to all licensees (such as establishment of radiation protection programs and the concept of as low as reasonably achievable [ALARA] exposure, dose limits for workers and members of the public, required surveys and monitoring, control and storage of licensed material, signage and posting of radiation areas, labeling radioactive material and handling of packages, and required records and reports). The purpose of the Part 20 regulations is to control the receipt, possession, use, transfer, and disposal of licensed material by any licensee in such

a manner that the total dose to an individual does not exceed the regulatory standards for protection against radiation. Excluded from the limits are doses from background radiation, exposure of patients to radiation for the purpose of medical diagnosis or therapy, exposure from individuals administered radioactive material and released in accordance with 10 CFR 35.75, and exposure from voluntary participation in medical research programs.

Part 30 Rules of General Applicability to Domestic Licensing of Byproduct Material.
Prescribes rules applicable to all persons in the United States governing the domestic licensing of byproduct material. These requirements must be met to obtain a license for medical use (10 CFR Part 35.18(a)(4)).

Part 35 Medical Use of Byproduct Material.
Contains requirements specific to medical use licensees, such as minimum training and experience criteria for authorized users, radiation safety officers, authorized nuclear pharmacists, and authorized medical physicists for knowledge and skills in radiation safety that are important to protect patients, the public, and workers in diagnostic and therapeutic medicine, and specific requirements for radiation health and safety from unsealed byproduct material that is administered to patients and human research subjects, including requirements that:

(1) Licensees supervise and instruct individuals in their radiation protection program in the applicable NRC regulations and conditions of the licenses to provide reasonable assurance of protection for health and safety of workers and the public, including patients;
(2) Patient dosages be accurately determined before patient administration and that instruments used to measure patient dosages are calibrated properly; and
(3) Syringes and vials that contain byproduct material for medical use are appropriately labeled to prevent administration of wrong dosages to patients.

4.2.1 Revisions to 10 CFR Part 35

The NRC has recently revised its regulations in 10 CFR Part 35, using a risk-informed and performance-based approach. The rule became effective on October 24, 2002, for NRC licensees; Agreement States have 3 years to comply with the revision. Highlights of the revised rule include:

(1) A new term, "medical event" (an event that meets the criteria in § 35.3045(a)), replaces the previous term "misadministration." A "medical event" involves a dose that exceeds 5 rem (0.05 Sv) effective dose equivalent (EDE), 50 rem (0.5 Sv) to an organ or tissue, or 50 rem (0.5 Sv) shallow-dose equivalent to the skin. The regulations continue to require that, when a medical event occurs, the licensee must notify the NRC, the referring physician, and the affected patient, unless the referring physician personally informs the licensee either that he or she will inform the individual or that, based on medical judgment, telling the individual would be harmful. As shown by the levels of radiation dose associated with common diagnostic radiopharmaceuticals in Table 2.1, "medical events" are extremely unlikely to occur as a result of any diagnostic nuclear medicine procedure.
(2) Some of the training and experience requirements for individuals performing diagnostic procedures using radioactive materials in unsealed form have been reduced. The training and experience requirements contained in Subpart J of the current regulation are also being retained for a 2-year period from the effective date of the revised rule; thus, before October 25, 2004, a licensee may comply with the appropriate training requirements either in Subpart J or in the revised requirements (10 CFR Part 35.10(c)).
(3) The revised rule contains a new requirement for reporting medical radiation exposure >5 rem (0.05 Sv) to an embryo/fetus (unless the dose was specifically approved, in advance, by the authorized user [§ 35.3047(a)]) or >5 rem (0.05 Sv) total EDE to a nursing child or that

has resulted in unintended permanent functional damage to an organ or a physiological system of the child (§ 35.3047(b)). The regulatory limit for the dose to an embryo, fetus, or nursing child is 0.5 rem (5 mSv). As discussed in Chapter 2, a dose >5 rem to an embryo/fetus or breast feeding infant is highly unlikely as a result of diagnostic nuclear medicine procedures. If a lactating woman undergoes a diagnostic nuclear medicine procedure, the authorized user physician should discuss breast feeding options (interruption or cessation) and instruct the patient, if appropriate, on ways to minimize radiation exposure to the infant.

(4) When a requirement in the revised Part 35 differs from the requirement in an existing license condition, the requirement in revised Part 35 will govern (10 CFR 35.10(e)). This paragraph primarily applies to those licensees that committed to follow the procedures in Regulatory Guide 10.8, *Guide for the Preparation of Applications for Medical Use Programs* (superceded by the rule and implementing guidance). For example, most licensees have committed to calibrate their dose calibrators using the procedures in Regulatory Guide 10.8, Appendix C, *Model Procedure for Calibrating Dose Calibrator.* These procedures are very prescriptive, and the revised Part 35.60(b) requires only that licensees calibrate instruments used to measure activity dosages in accordance with nationally recognized standards or the manufacturer's instructions.

4.2.2 Rationale for Changes

The revised Part 35 generally has achieved a significant reduction in the regulatory burden associated with diagnostic nuclear medicine. The NRC believes that the regulatory burden of the revised rule is commensurate with the low risk of adverse impact on health and safety from these diagnostic procedures and that further reduction of regulatory burden has the potential to increase the risk to public health and safety. The underlying premise of NRC regulations is that authorized user physicians will understand radiation safety principles and practices and will make decisions that are in the best interests of their patients. Clearly, regulations will not prevent all unintended exposures, but the requirements serve to remind licensees that they have certain responsibilities and need to implement a series of checks and balances to ensure the security and safe use of licensed material. 10 CFR Part 35 contains requirements for diagnostic and therapeutic uses of byproduct material (the latter therapy applications are not confined to nuclear medicine but also are used in brachytherapy, remote afterloaders, teletherapy units, and gamma stereotactic radiosurgery units). It is important to provide clear guidance to diagnostic nuclear medicine practitioners in the associated licensing guidance and also to ensure that the licensing guidance reflects regulatory requirements. This is the raison d'être of this section of this book—to provide a stand-alone document useful to diagnostic nuclear medicine practitioners.

It must be understood that Part 35 cannot be looked at in isolation. The Commission's regulatory framework consists of several interrelated documents, including Title 10 of the Code of Federal Regulations (especially Parts 19, 20, and 30), statements of policy, and licensing and inspection guidance. The implementation of the revised Part 35 through licensing and inspection should both protect public health and safety and provide effective regulation that does not add unnecessary regulatory burden in a "risk-informed, performance-based" manner. Licensees, by definition, have obtained NRC permission to use byproduct materials for medical use. Attached to this permission is the required commitment to radiation protection policies and implementing procedures. The policies and procedures in this book will assist diagnostic nuclear medicine licensees in complying with the rule. Chapter 9 contains suggested procedures for compliance. Licensees should consider their own prior experience and review of their facilities' established radiation protection programs when adopting these suggested procedures.

Because the NRC has also committed to a risk-informed, performance-based approach to inspection, which will focus on outcomes and not procedures (i.e., the inspections will directly deal with NRC requirements), the NRC regulations and suggested operating policies and procedures in this book should not be used as the primary inspection criteria, unless there is a performance failure.

The NRC intends to ask the following three questions when evaluating licensee errors:

(1) What could happen?
(2) How likely is it?
(3) What are the consequences?

Procedural omissions or lapses in teaching or supervision of nuclear medicine technologists in these procedures are not the reasons for every misstep. In spite of written policies and procedures, accidents may happen. However, unless safety is compromised, this should not elicit a regulatory concern unless there is a problem with licensee performance outcomes.

4.3 Medical Use Policy Statement

In August 2000, the NRC published (*Fed Reg.* August 3, 2000; 65:47654–47660) a revision to its 1979 policy statement on the medical use of byproduct material.

The following is the Medical Use Policy Statement to guide NRC's future regulation of the medical use of byproduct material:

(1) NRC will continue to regulate the uses of radionuclides in medicine as necessary to provide for the radiation safety of workers and the general public.
(2) NRC will not intrude into medical judgments affecting patients, except as necessary to provide for the radiation safety of workers and the general public.
(3) NRC will, when justified by the risk to patients, regulate the radiation safety of patients primarily to assure that the use of radionuclides is in accordance with the physician's directions.
(4) NRC, in developing a specific regulatory approach, will consider industry and professional standards that define acceptable approaches of achieving radiation safety.

5 Nuclear Regulatory Commission and Agreement States

Certain states, called Agreement States, have entered into regulatory contracts (agreements) with the Nuclear Regulatory Commission (NRC) that give them the authority to license and inspect byproduct, source, or special nuclear material used or possessed within their borders. Except for the use of the latter special radioactive materials, states have the responsibility for public health and safety for all other applications of ionizing radiation in medicine. The Atomic Energy Act was revised in 1959 to establish the Agreement State program, whereby Atomic Energy Commission responsibilities for health and safety could be delegated to a state. In 1962, Kentucky became the first Agreement State. There are currently 32 Agreement States and 18 non-Agreement or NRC States (Minnesota, Pennsylvania, and Wisconsin have filed letters of intent to become Agreement States). It should be noted that nuclear materials in federal agencies, such as Veterans Affairs hospitals, are regulated by the NRC regardless of location.

The NRC is responsible for regulating the use of:

(1) Source material (uranium and thorium) and associated processing waste;

(2) Special nuclear material (enriched uranium and plutonium); and

(3) Byproduct material (reactor-produced).

The States regulate other radiation sources:

(1) Naturally occurring radioactive material (radium and radon);

(2) Particle accelerator–produced radioactive material (^{18}F, ^{57}Co, ^{67}Ga, ^{111}In, ^{123}I, ^{201}Tl); and

(3) Radiation-producing machines.

Thus, as an example, the States, not the NRC, regulate the use of positron emission tomographic radiopharmaceuticals. For NRC licensees, these are considered unlicensed materials. It should be noted that the purpose of the Part 20 regulations, pursuant to § 20.1001(b), is to limit the total dose to an individual not only from licensed radioactive material but also from unlicensed material and from radiation sources other than background radiation. The Conference of Radiation Control Program Directors (CRCPD), established in 1968, is a voluntary network of state and local government officials responsible for radiation regulation and enforcement; it has no regulatory authority. The CRCPD creates *Suggested State Regulations for Control of Radiation.* Most state radiation protection programs are based on these suggested guidelines. Part G, *Use of Radionuclides in the Healing Arts,* is the medical regulatory section. Agreement States also belong to the Organization of Agreement States.

It is important to point out that the NRC's risk-informed, performance-based approach to licensing and, more important, to inspection may not occur in all Agreement States. Some states may use licensee-adopted procedural implementations as standards to inspect against. Model procedures in this book are merely samples, not minimum standards, and should not replace the regulations. The primary measure of a licensee's compliance and safe use of licensed materials should be their performance outcomes, which are direct and objective measures of safety. Inspecting against model procedures only is an indirect and subjective approach using "surrogates" for safety. Agreement State guidance documents can be more restrictive than those of the NRC and thus stay prescriptive rather than participate in the transition to a risk-informed, performance-based approach. Licensees in these states should monitor the activities of their rulemaking bodies.

6

Nuclear Regulatory Commission Licenses for Medical Use

The Nuclear Regulatory Commission (NRC) issues three types of licenses for the use of byproduct material in medical practices and facilities:

(1) General in vitro license;

(2) Specific license of limited scope; and

(3) Specific license of broad scope.

The license typically obtained for diagnostic nuclear medicine purposes is the specific license of limited scope. The NRC issues this type of license to private or group medical practices and to medical institutions. Individual physicians or physician groups located within a licensed medical facility may not apply for a separate license (10 CFR 30.33(a)(2) refers to the applicant's facilities). The facility's management must sign the license application and has authority for the radiation protection program. The radiation safety officer is appointed by management and must accept, in writing, responsibility for implementing the radiation protection program. The authorized user physician(s) is specifically listed in the license.

Medical institutions that provide patient care and conduct research programs that use byproduct materials for in vitro, animal, and medical procedures may request a specific license of broad scope in accordance with 10 CFR Part 33, *Specific Domestic Licenses of Broad Scope for Byproduct Material.* These types of institutions generally deal with higher risk procedures, such as therapeutic administrations with sealed sources in devices, than are encountered in diagnostic nuclear medicine and have a well-staffed radiation safety office for the purpose of implementing the additional necessary radiation protection–related requirements unique to higher risk procedures.

7

Revised Part 35 Requirements Applicable to Diagnostic Nuclear Medicine

The revised 10 CFR Part 35 does not use or define the term "diagnostic nuclear medicine." Medical uses are categorized according to the written directive requirement (§ 35.40 and § 35.41) and physical form of byproduct material (unsealed material or sealed sources). A written directive is a written order for the administration of byproduct material to a specific patient or human research subject and is required before the administration of ^{131}I-sodium iodide in an amount >30µCi (1.11 MBq) or any therapeutic dosage of any other unsealed byproduct material. The use of ^{131}I-sodium iodide in amounts >30 µCi requires a written directive and is included, therefore, with therapeutic uses. Written directives are generally not necessary in diagnostic nuclear medicine, because they are required only for radionuclide therapy and for the administration of ^{131}I-sodium iodide in amounts >30 µCi (1.11 MBq). This activity of ^{131}I is typically not exceeded when performing thyroid uptake measurements. The 30-µCi limit for ^{131}I applies only to Na^{131}I. Diagnostic studies with other ^{131}I-labeled radiopharmaceuticals (e.g., ^{131}I-metaiodobenzylguanadine, ^{131}I-hippuran, ^{131}I-iodocholesterol) may be performed with activities >30 µCi without the need for a written directive.

Diagnostic nuclear medicine procedures are understood to be described or referenced in Subpart D, *Unsealed Byproduct Material—Written Directive Not Required,* specifically in sections:

10 CFR 35.100 Use of unsealed byproduct material for uptake, dilution, and excretion studies for which a written directive is not required.

Although most facilities performing diagnostic nuclear medicine procedures will apply for § 35.200 status, it is recognized that some facilities may request § 35.100 status. § 35.100 governs a more limited set of medical procedures and requires a shorter training program for workers.

10 CFR 35.200 Use of unsealed byproduct material for imaging and localization studies for which a written directive is not required.

A licensee authorized to use the procedures in 10 CFR 35.200 also will be able to perform the procedures in § 35.100, such as thyroid uptakes (as noted above, the reverse is not true because of increased requirements for training and experience for § 35.200 procedures), provided the license includes authorization for parts 100 and 200. This is applicable for all diagnostic nuclear medicine licensees using § 35.200 materials. It must be noted that licensees performing thyroid scintigraphy or extended scintigraphy for differentiated thyroid cancer will administer Na^{131}I in amounts >30 µCi (1.11 MBq), which require a written directive, and are therefore subject to the requirements in 10 CFR 35.300, *Use of unsealed byproduct material for which a written directive is required.* (These are additional requirements that will not be detailed here.) For example, if licensees intend to use >30 µCi (1.11 MBq) Na^{131}I for diagnostic purposes (typically scanning doses of 2–5 mCi [74–185 MBq] are used), they are required to have additional training and experience, use written directives, perform additional radiation surveys, and may be required to institute a bioassay program.

7.1 Part 35 Subparts

The revised Part 35 rule is organized into Subparts A though N. The requirements for diagnostic and therapeutic medicine are intermingled. As a first step in making these requirements more "user-friendly," they were reviewed and only those requirements applicable to diagnostic nuclear medicine uses of § 35.100 and § 35.200 materials were identified here . All of these requirements will be covered in Chapters 8 and 9.

Subpart A General Information

35.2 Definitions.

35.5 Maintenance of records.

35.6 Provisions for research involving human subjects.

35.7 Food and Drug Administration, other federal, and state requirements.

35.10 Implementation.

35.11 License required.

35.12 Application for license, amendment, or renewal.

35.13 License amendments.

35.14 Notifications.

35.18 License issuance.

35.19 Specific exemptions.

Subpart B General Administrative Requirements

35.24 Authority and responsibilities for the radiation protection program.

35.26 Radiation protection program changes.

35.27 Supervision.

35.50 Training for radiation safety officer.

35.51 Training for an authorized medical physicist.

35.55 Training for an authorized nuclear pharmacist.

35.57 Training for experienced Radiation Safety Officer, teletherapy or medical physicist, authorized user, and nuclear pharmacist.

35.59 Recentness of training.

Subpart C General Technical Requirements

35.60 Possession, use, calibration, and check of instruments to measure the activity of unsealed byproduct material.

35.61 Calibration of survey instruments.

35.63 Determination of dosages of unsealed byproduct material for medical use.

35.65 Authorization for calibration, transmission, and reference sources.

35.67 Requirements for possession of sealed sources and brachytherapy sources.

35.69 Labeling of vials and syringes.

35.75 Release of individuals containing unsealed byproduct material or implants containing byproduct material.

35.80 Provision of mobile medical service.

35.92 Decay-in-storage.

Subpart D Unsealed Byproduct Material. Written Directive Not Required

35.100 Use of unsealed byproduct material for uptake, dilution, and excretion studies for which a written directive is not required.

35.190 Training for uptake, dilution, and excretion studies.

35.200 Use of unsealed byproduct material for imaging and localization studies for which a written directive is not required.

35.204 Permissible ^{99}Mo concentration.

35.290 Training for imaging and localization studies.

Subpart J Training and Experience Requirements (Retained as part of the regulation for 2 years)

35.900 Radiation safety officer.

35.910 Training for uptake, dilution, and excretion studies.

35.920 Training for imaging and localization studies.

35.961 Training for an authorized medical physicist.

35.980 Training for an authorized nuclear pharmacist.

35.981 Training for experienced nuclear pharmacists.

Subpart L Records

35.2024 Records of authority and responsibilities for radiation protection program.

35.2026 Records of radiation protection program changes.

35.2060 Records of calibrations of instruments used to measure the activity of unsealed byproduct materials.

35.2061 Records of radiation survey instrument calibrations.

35.2063 Records of dosages of unsealed byproduct material for medical use.

35.2067 Records of leaks tests and inventory of sealed sources and brachytherapy sources.

35.2080 Records of mobile medical services.

35.2092 Records of decay-in-storage.

35.2204 Records of ^{99}Mo concentrations.

Subpart M Reports

35.3045 Report and notification of a medical event.

35.3047 Report and notification of a dose to an embryo/fetus or a nursing child.

35.3067 Report of a leaking source.

Subpart N Enforcement

35.4001 Violations.

35.4002 Criminal penalties.

8

Training and Experience Requirements for Diagnostic Nuclear Medicine

It is important to the radiation safety of workers and the public, including patients, to designate certain individuals who have adequate training and experience in radiation safety principles as applied to diagnostic nuclear medicine. This reduces unnecessary radiation exposure while obtaining diagnostic information that will benefit the patient. Training and experience requirements to demonstrate sufficient knowledge and skills in radiation protection practices and procedures are essential for identifying individuals who may work as:

(1) Authorized user physician (AU);
(2) Radiation safety officer (RSO);
(3) Authorized nuclear pharmacist (ANP); and
(4) Authorized medical physicist (AMP).

The high level of protection afforded to patients, workers, and the public by the practice of diagnostic nuclear medicine is in part the result of the training and experience of these authorized individuals. Usually, these authorized individuals supervise other workers who are involved in medical use. They must direct these supervised individuals to ensure that unsealed byproduct material is handled safely. Many of these supervised individuals are nuclear medicine technologists, but no Nuclear Regulatory Commission (NRC) requirements specify their training and experience. Nationally approved training programs for nuclear medicine technologists have been in existence for many years. In some states, students must pass an examination as a certified nuclear medicine technologist in order to be licensed to practice in that state.

The NRC requires that an applicant/licensee be "qualified by training and experience to use licensed materials for the purposes requested in such a manner as to protect health and minimize danger to life or property" (§ 30.33). Diagnostic nuclear medicine purposes are generally for the use of unsealed byproduct material for which a written directive is not required, and these uses are covered by 10 CFR 35.100 and 35.200, as previously discussed. Almost all diagnostic nuclear medicine licensees perform the studies in 10 CFR 35.200 and may use any unsealed byproduct material not requiring a written directive prepared for medical use that is:

(1) Obtained from a manufacturer or preparer that is appropriately licensed by NRC or equivalent Agreement State requirements;
(2) Prepared by an ANP, a physician who is an AU and who meets the requirements in § 35.290, § 35.390, or an individual under the supervision of either as specified in § 35.27;
(3) Obtained from and prepared by an NRC or Agreement State licensee for use in research in accordance with a Radioactive Drug Research Committee (RDRC)–approved protocol or an Investigational New Drug (IND) protocol accepted by the U.S. Food and Drug Administration; or
(4) Prepared by a licensee for use in research in accordance with an RDRC-approved application or an IND protocol accepted by the FDA.

The NRC training and experience requirements for AUs involved with § 35.200 materials and procedures and RSOs are detailed here. Because most diagnostic nuclear medicine facilities do not employ ANPs or AMPs, their training and experience requirements are not included. The interested reader is referred to the pertinent regulations (ANP: § 35.55, § 35.59, § 35.980, § 35.981; AMP: § 35.51, § 35.59, § 35.961).

8.1 Revised Requirements

The training and experience requirements in the revised Part 35 have been changed. In addition to the reduced hours necessary for an AU, the new rule basically requires that AUs and RSOs meet either of the following two criteria:

(1) Certification by a specialty board whose certification process includes stated requirements and whose certification has been recognized by the NRC or an Agreement State; or
(2) Completion of specified hours of didactic training and work experience under an AU or RSO; and
(3) Written certification signed by a preceptor AU or RSO.

Another route is available for RSOs according to § 35.50. An RSO can be an individual who is identified as an AU (or AMP or ANP) on the licensee's license and has experience with the radiation safety aspects of similar types of use of byproduct material for which the individual has RSO responsibilities.

Previously, AUs and RSOs were required to be either certified by certain recognized specialty boards or obtain the requisite training and experience without written certification by a preceptor. As of October 2002, with the exception of the Certification Board of Nuclear Cardiology, no certifying boards are recognized by the NRC. The revised rule therefore includes a 2-year transition period for training and experience requirements. During this time the current or revised requirements may be used. According to 10 CFR Part 35.10, before October 25, 2004, a licensee can satisfy the training requirements for an RSO and AU by complying with either:

(1) The appropriate training requirements in subpart J (§ 35.900, § 35.910,§ 35.920); or
(2) The appropriate training requirements in § 35.50, § 35.57, § 35.59, § 35.190, and/or § 35.290.

Subpart J of Part 35 has been retained for a 2-year period.

8.1.1 Authorized User Physician

10 CFR 35.290 Training for imaging and localization studies.

To become an AU of unsealed byproduct material for the uses authorized under § 35.200 a physician must meet one of the following criteria (except as provided in § 35.57):

(1) Certification by a medical specialty board whose certification process includes all of the requirements in item 2 and whose certification has been recognized by the Commission or an Agreement State.
(2) Completion of 700 hours of training and experience including all of the following:
  a. Classroom and laboratory training in:
    i. Radiation physics and instrumentation;
    ii. Radiation protection;
    iii. Mathematics pertaining to use and measurements of radioactivity;
    iv. Chemistry of byproduct material for medical use; and
    v. Radiation biology.
  b. Work experience under supervision of AU who meets requirements in § 35.290, § 35.390, or equivalent Agreement State requirements, involving:
    i. Ordering, receiving, and unpacking radioactive materials safely and performing related radiation surveys;
    ii. Calibrating instruments used to determine the activity of dosages and performing checks for proper operation of survey meters;
    iii. Calculating, measuring, and safely preparing patient or human research subject dosages;
    iv. Using administrative controls to prevent medical events;
    v. Using procedures to safely contain spills and using proper decontamination procedures;
    vi. Administering dosages of radioactive drugs to patients or human research subjects; and
    vii. Eluting generator systems appropriate for preparation of radioactive drugs for imaging and localization studies, measuring and testing the eluate for radionuclidic purity, and processing eluate with reagent kits to prepare labeled radioactive drugs.
  c. Obtained written certification, signed by a preceptor AU who meets requirements in § 35.290, § 35.390, or equivalent Agreement State requirements, that the individual has satisfactorily completed the requirements in

2(a) and 2(b) and has achieved a level of competency sufficient to function independently as an AU for the medical uses authorized under § 35.100 and § 35.200.

(Note: The preceptor must certify the "competency" of the individual, but the requirements do not state how competency should be determined. This places a high degree of responsibility on the preceptor. The NRC does not believe that this is an undue burden but, instead, that it demonstrates a high degree of confidence in the preceptor. Further, the NRC believes that judgments of competency in training and experience are consistent with the duties of individuals who direct training programs or provide training.)

10 CFR 35.920 Training for imaging and localization studies. (Subpart J; retained for 2 years)

To become an AU of radiopharmaceuticals, generators, or reagent kits for imaging and localization studies, a physician must meet one of the following criteria (except as provided in § 35.57):

(1) Certification by any of the following:
  a. American Board of Nuclear Medicine (in nuclear medicine);
  b. American Board of Radiology (in diagnostic radiology);
  c. American Osteopathic Board of Radiology (in diagnostic radiology or radiology);
  d. Royal College of Physicians and Surgeons of Canada (in nuclear medicine); or
  e. American Osteopathic Board of Nuclear Medicine (in nuclear medicine).

(2) Completion of training and experience, including all of the following:
  a. 200 hours of classroom and laboratory training in:
    i. Radiation physics and instrumentation;
    ii. Radiation protection;
    iii. Mathematics pertaining to use and measurements of radioactivity;
    iv. Radiopharmaceutical chemistry; and
    v. Radiation biology.
  b. 500 hours of supervised work experience under supervision of an AU in:
    i. Ordering, receiving, and unpacking of radioactive materials safely and performing related radiation surveys;
    ii. Calibrating dose calibrators and diagnostic instruments and performing checks for proper operation of survey meters;
    iii. Calculating, measuring, and safely preparing patient or human research subject dosages;
    iv. Using administrative controls to prevent medical events;
    v. Using procedures to safely contain spills and using proper decontamination procedures; and
    vi. Eluting ^{99m}Tc from generators, testing for ^{99}Mo and alumina contamination, and preparing ^{99m}Tc-labeled agents.
  c. 500 hours of supervised clinical experience under supervision of an AU in:
    i. Examining patients/research subjects and reviewing case histories to determine their suitability for nuclear medicine diagnostic procedures;
    ii. Selecting suitable radiopharmaceuticals and calculating and measuring the dosages;
    iii. Administering patient or human research subject dosages and using syringe radiation shields;
    iv. Reviewing radiopharmaceutical test results with AU; and
    v. Performing patient/research subject follow-up.

(3) Successful completion of a 6-month training program in nuclear medicine approved by the Accreditation Council for Graduate Medical Education that included all requirements in item 2.

10 CFR 35.57 Training for experienced Radiation Safety Officer, teletherapy or medical physicist, authorized user, and nuclear pharmacist.

Physicians identified as AUs for the medical use of byproduct material on a license issued by the Commission or Agreement State, a permit issued by a Commission master material licensee, a permit issued by a Commission or Agreement State broad scope licensee, or a permit issued by a Commission master material license broad scope permittee before October 24, 2002, who perform only those medical uses for which they were authorized on that date need not comply with the training requirements of § 35.290.

10 CFR 35.59 Recentness of training.
The training and experience specified in § 35.290 and § 35.920 must have been obtained within the 7 years preceding the date of application or the individual must have had related continuing education and experience since the required training and experience were completed.

8.1.2 Radiation Safety Officer

10 CFR 35.50 Training for Radiation Safety Officer.
To become an RSO, an individual must meet one of the following criteria (except as provided in § 35.57):

(1) Certification by a specialty board whose certification process includes all of the requirements in item 2 and whose certification has been recognized by the Commission or an Agreement State.

(2) Completion of training and experience, including all of the following:

a. 200 hours of didactic training in:
  i. Radiation physics and instrumentation;
  ii. Radiation protection;
  iii. Mathematics pertaining to use and measurements of radioactivity;
  iv. Radiation biology; and
  v. Radiation dosimetry.

b. One year of full-time radiation safety experience under supervision of individual identified as RSO on Commission or Agreement State license or permit issued by a Commission master material licensee that authorizes similar type of use of byproduct material involving:
  i. Shipping, receiving, and performing related radiation surveys;
  ii. Using and performing checks for proper operation of instruments used to determine activity of dosages, survey meters, and instruments used to measure radionuclides;
  iii. Securing and controlling byproduct material;
  iv. Using administrative controls to avoid mistakes in the administration of byproduct material;
  v. Using procedures to prevent or minimize radioactive contamination and using proper decontamination procedures;
  vi. Using emergency procedures to control byproduct material; and
  vii. Disposing of byproduct material.

c. Obtained written certification, signed by a preceptor RSO, that the individual has satisfactorily completed the requirements in 2(a) and 2(b) and has achieved a level of radiation safety knowledge sufficient to function independently as an RSO for a medical use licensee.

(3) Identification as an AU (or AMP or ANP) on licensee's license and experience with the radiation safety aspects of similar types of use of byproduct material for which the individual has RSO responsibilities.

10 CFR 35.900 Radiation Safety Officer. (Subpart J; retained for 2 years)
To become an RSO, an individual must meet one of the following criteria (except as provided in § 35.57):

(1) Certification by any of the following:
  a. American Board of Health Physics in comprehensive health physics;
  b. American Board of Radiology;
  c. American Board of Nuclear Medicine;
  d. American Board of Science in Nuclear Medicine;
  e. Board of Pharmaceutical Specialties in nuclear pharmacy;
  f. American Board of Medical Physics in radiation oncology physics;
  g. Royal College of Physicians and Surgeons of Canada in nuclear medicine;
  h. American Osteopathic Board Radiology; or
  i. American Osteopathic Board of Nuclear Medicine

(2) Completion of training and experience, including all of the following:

a. 200 hours of classroom and laboratory training in:
   i. Radiation physics and instrumentation;
   ii. Radiation protection;
   iii. Mathematics pertaining to use and measurements of radioactivity;
   iv. Radiation biology; and
   v. Radiopharmaceutical chemistry.
b. One year of full-time experience as a radiation safety technologist at a medical institution under supervision of individual identified as RSO on NRC or Agreement State license that authorizes the medical use of byproduct material.

(3) Identification as an AU on licensee's license.

10 CFR 35.57 Training for experienced Radiation Safety Officer, teletherapy or medical physicist, authorized user, and nuclear pharmacist.

An individual identified as an RSO on a Commission or Agreement State license or a permit issued by a Commission or Agreement State broad scope licensee or master material license permit or by a master material license permittee of broad scope before October 24, 2002, need not comply with the training requirements of § 35.50.

10 CFR 35.59 Recentness of training.

The training and experience specified in § 35.50 and § 35.900 must have been obtained within the 7 years preceding the date of application or the individual must have had related continuing education and experience since the original training and experience were completed.

Regulatory Issues at a Glance: Training and Experience

Authorized user

Radiation safety officer

(Authorized nuclear pharmacist and authorized medical physicist)

(Experienced authorized user, authorized nuclear pharmacist, and authorized medical physicist)

Recentness of training

9

Radiation Protection Program

Key elements of a radiation protection program include responsibility, accountability, and authority. At the heart of any such program is the training and experience of the personnel involved, as addressed previously in Chapter 8.

Each area in the following chapter will provide:

(1) All pertinent Nuclear Regulatory Commission (NRC) requirements for the medical use of byproduct material in the practice of diagnostic nuclear medicine. These have been summarized in the interest of space; licensees should read the actual regulations. It should be noted that these are NRC regulations and, as such, may not apply in Agreement States. Nuclear medicine practitioners in Agreement States must contact their respective rulemaking bodies.

(2) A discussion of the requirements;

(3) Suggested procedures for compliance; and

(4) Quick-reference boxes with pertinent subtopics and relevant regulations.

Radiation Protection Program (General)

Pertinent regulations:

10 CFR 19.11	Posting of notices to workers.
10 CFR 19.31	Application for exemptions.
10 CFR 20.1101	Radiation protection programs.
10 CFR 20.2301	Applications for exemptions.
10 CFR 20.2302	Additional requirements.
10 CFR 30.11	Specific exemptions.
10 CFR 30.33	General requirements for issuance of specific licenses.
10 CFR 30.34	Terms and conditions of licenses.
10 CFR 35.19	Specific exemptions.
10 CFR 35.24	Authority and responsibilities for the radiation protection program.
10 CFR 35.26	Radiation protection program changes.

The complete text of these regulations can be accessed online through the NRC electronic reading room at www.nrc.gov.

9.1 Radiation Protection Program (General)

9.1.1 Pertinent Regulations

10 CFR 19.11 Posting of notices to workers.

Each licensee must post current copies of the operating procedures applicable to licensed activities.

10 CFR 19.31 Application for exemptions.

The Commission, upon application by any licensee or upon its own initiative, may grant such exemptions from the Part 19 requirements as it determines are authorized by law and will not result in undue hazard to life or property.

10 CFR 20.1101 Radiation protection programs.

Each licensee must develop, document, and implement a radiation protection program commensurate with the scope and extent of licensed activities and sufficient to ensure compliance with the requirements in Part 20.

The licensee must use, to the extent practical, procedures and engineering controls based upon sound radiation protection principles to achieve occupational doses and doses to members of the public that are as low as reasonably achievable (ALARA).

The licensee must periodically (at least annually) review the radiation protection program content and implementation.

10 CFR 20.2301 Applications for exemptions.

The Commission, upon application by a licensee or upon its own initiative, may grant an exemption from the Part 20 requirements if it determines the exemption is authorized by law and would not result in undue hazard to life or property.

10 CFR 20.2302 Additional requirements.

The Commission, by rule, regulation, or order, may

impose requirements on a licensee, in addition to those established in the Part 20 regulations, as it deems appropriate or necessary to protect health or to minimize danger to life or property.

10 CFR 30.11 Specific exemptions.

The Commission, upon application of any interested person or upon its own initiative, may grant such exemptions from the requirements in Part 30 and Parts 31–36 and 39 as it determines are authorized by law and will not endanger life or property or the common defense and security and are otherwise in the public interest.

10 CFR 30.33 General requirements for issuance of specific licenses.

An application for a specific license will be approved if the applicant's proposed equipment and facilities are adequate to protect health and minimize danger to life or property.

10 CFR 30.34 Terms and conditions of licenses.

Section (e) states that the Commission may incorporate in any license issued pursuant to the regulations, additional requirements and conditions it deems appropriate or necessary in order to:

(1) Promote common defense and security;

(2) Protect health or minimize danger to life or property;

(3) Protect restricted data; and

(4) Require such reports and the keeping of such records, and to provide for such inspections of activities under the license as may be necessary or appropriate to effectuate the purposes of the Act and regulations thereunder.

10 CFR 35.19 Specific exemptions.

The Commission, upon application of any interested person or upon its own initiative, may grant exemptions from the Part 35 regulations that it determines are authorized by law and will not endanger life or property or the common defense and security and are otherwise in the public interest.

10 CFR 35.24 Authority and responsibilities for the radiation protection program.

In addition to the radiation protection program requirements of § 20.1101, a licensee's management must approve in writing radiation protection program changes that do not require a license amendment and are permitted under § 35.26. A record of actions taken by the licensee's management must be retained in accordance with § 35.2024.

10 CFR 35.26 Radiation protection program changes.

A licensee may change its radiation protection program without Commission approval if:

(1) The revision is in compliance with the regulations and the license;

(2) The revision has been reviewed and approved by the radiation safety officer (RSO) and licensee management;

(3) The affected individuals are instructed on the revised program before the changes are implemented; and

(4) A record is kept of these changes in accordance with § 35.2026.

TABLE 9.1

Elements of a Radiation Protection Program

A radiation protection program should include operating policies and implementing procedures that address:

Occupational dose limits	Page 28
Dose limits for members of the public	Page 36
Minimization of contamination/spill procedures	Page 39
Material receipt and accountability/ordering, receiving, and opening packages	Page 41
Radiation surveys and calibration of survey instruments	Page 43
Caution signs and posting requirements	Page 47
Labeling containers, vials, and syringes	Page 49
Determining patient dosages	Page 50
Sealed source inventory and leak testing	Page 52
Waste disposal and decay-in-storage	Page 53
Records	Page 54
Reports	Page 57
Safety instruction for workers	Page 60
Audit program	Page 62
Mobile diagnostic nuclear medicine services (if applicable)	Page 62

9.1.2 Discussion of the Requirements

Licensees must document their radiation protection programs. The extent of the program depends on the magnitude and complexity of the licensed activity and on the degree of risk to workers and the public. Written procedures have been the principal method by which diagnostic nuclear medicine licensees have established methods and processes to ensure proper and consistent implementation of their programs. Licensees must have a radiation protection program in place that contains operating policies and implementing procedures to ensure the security and safe use of unsealed byproduct material in diagnostic nuclear medicine, from the time it arrives at the licensee's facility until it is used, transferred, and/or disposed. Although individual responsibility cannot be underestimated, providing for the safe use of radioactive materials is a management responsibility. It is crucial, therefore, that management recognize the importance of the overall radiation protection program. Essential elements in such a program are listed in Table 9.1.

Licensees must develop, implement, and maintain specific policies and operating procedures in each area to ensure that their radiation protection programs are in compliance with the applicable regulations. Each licensee is required to use reasonable practices and controls to strive to maintain doses to workers and the public that are ALARA. The licensee must incorporate measures to track and, if necessary, reduce these exposures. All licensees must keep records of their radiation protection programs and audits and reviews. Records of any program changes also must be maintained. It should be noted that most diagnostic nuclear medicine licensees (i.e., those diagnostic practices not located in a medical institution with a broad scope license) are not required to have a radiation safety committee (§ 35.24(f)). Nevertheless, the licensee is required to review the radiation protection program at least annually. The Commission can also impose additional requirements on a licensee as it deems appropriate (§ 20.2302 and § 30.34(e)).

Under the NRC's new risk-informed, performance-based approach to regulation, the continued need for some of these procedures should be based on the diagnostic nuclear medicine licensee's own previous experience. One example would be in the review of workers' radiation dose histories obtained during the required radiation protection program review or at any other time. The purpose of the radiation protection program review is to cover procedural compliance, technical adequacy, implementation, and effectiveness. Lessons learned and suggested improvements from these reviews should be considered for program changes. Historically, the extremely low radiation risk associated with levels of radioactivity used in diagnostic nuclear medicine has been such that no cases of demonstrable harm to workers or to public health and safety have been documented.

It should be anticipated, therefore, that some of the suggested procedures for compliance discussed in this chapter could potentially be revised or even eliminated. However, vigilance should be maintained to ensure that current programs continue to meet regulatory requirements. Any changes must be reviewed and approved by the RSO and licensee management. All affected individuals also must be instructed on any revised program; there is no need for NRC approval in the form of a license amendment (§ 35.26). In addition, the NRC is willing to consider an application for an exemption from the requirements in Part 19 (§19.31), Part 20 (§ 20.2301), Part 30 (§ 30.11), or Part 35 (§ 35.19). For example, based on periodic reviews of performance of the licensee's own prior experience, a licensee may determine that exemption from certain requirements would not compromise public health and safety. In this case, the licensee should apply to the NRC for relief from this regulatory burden. The NRC addresses requests on a case-by-case basis. A request for exemption may or may not be granted based on the specifics of the request. Of course, new applicants should implement all the suggested procedures as written until they can demonstrate that they may be revised or are no longer necessary to ensure compliance with the regulations.

Although it has been stated previously, it is important to remember that the suggested implementing procedures for the radiation protection program in this chapter are merely samples and not minimum standards or "best practices." Despite these written procedures, accidents may occur. Procedural omissions are not the reason for every misstep; human error, for example, may be involved. Nevertheless, the radiation protection program should be able to identify program weaknesses and develop corrective action.

9.1.3 Suggested Procedures for Compliance

The following general procedures may be included in any radiation protection program designed to promote the security and safe use of byproduct materials in diagnostic nuclear medicine:

(1) Wear laboratory coats in areas where radioactive materials are present.
(2) Wear disposable gloves at all times when handling radioactive materials.
(3) Monitor hands and body for radioactive contamination before leaving the area.
(4) Use syringe and vial shields as necessary.
(5) Do not eat, drink, smoke, apply cosmetics, or store food in any area where licensed material is stored or used.
(6) If required, wear personnel monitoring devices (e.g., whole body and/or ring badge) at all times when in areas where radioactive materials are used or stored. When not being worn to monitor occupational dose, these devices must be stored in a low-background area.
(7) Never pipette by mouth.
(8) Dispose of radioactive waste only in designated, labeled, and properly shielded receptacles located in a secured (e.g., locked) area.
(9) Appropriately label all containers, vials, and syringes containing radioactive materials. When not in use, place these in shielded containers (e.g., lead pigs) or behind appropriate lead shielding in a secured area if not under constant surveillance and control.
(10) Store all sealed sources (e.g., flood sources and dose calibrator check sources, if needed) in shielded containers in a secured area when not in use.
(11) Before administering dosages to patients, determine and record activity (based on either decay correction or dose calibrator measurement, whichever method is selected for use).
(12) Know what steps to take and who to contact (e.g., radiation safety officer) in the event of radiation incidents (such as unsealed material spills or a leaking sealed source), improper operation of radiation safety equipment, or theft/loss of licensed material.

Regulatory Issues at a Glance: Radiation Protection Program (General)

- Radiation protection policies and implementing procedures
- Authority and responsibilities
- ALARA policy
- Periodic reviews of program
- Program changes
- Exemptions

(13) To minimize spread of radioactive contamination and facilitate decontamination, use absorbent paper in areas where liquid licensed materials are prepared or used (e.g., cover all areas of use in the hot lab).

The radiation protection program also must include the functional areas discussed in 9.2–9.16. Suggested procedures, especially for new applicants and for those licensees that have recently undergone a major personnel or physical plant change, are provided here.

9.2 Occupational Dose Limits

9.2.1 Pertinent Regulations

10 CFR 19.13 Notifications and reports to individuals. Workers who are required to be monitored must be advised of their dose limits annually by licensees.

10 CFR 20.1201 Occupational dose limits for adults. Licensee must control occupational dose to adults to the following annual limits:

(1) The more limiting of:
  a. 5 rem (0.05 Sv)—total effective dose equivalent (TEDE); or
  b. 50 rem (0.5 Sv)—sum of deep-dose equivalent (DDE) and committed dose equivalent to any organ or tissue (other than lens of the eye).
(2) 15 rem (0.15 Sv)—lens dose equivalent (LDE).
(3) 50 rem (0.5 Sv)—shallow-dose equivalent (SDE) to skin or any extremity.

The DDE and SDE must be assigned for the part of the body receiving the highest exposure. If the individual monitoring device was not in the region of highest potential exposure or results of monitoring are unavailable, the required doses may be assessed from surveys or other radiation measurements.

Occupational Dose Limits

Pertinent regulations:

10 CFR 19.13	Notifications and reports to individuals.
10 CFR 20.1201	Occupational dose limits for adults.
10 CFR 20.1202	Compliance with requirements for summation of external and internal doses.
10 CFR 20.1203	Determination of external dose from airborne radioactive material.
10 CFR 20.1204	Determination of internal exposure.
10 CFR 20.1207	Occupational dose limits for minors.
10 CFR 20.1208	Dose to an embryo/fetus.
10 CFR 20.1501	General.
10 CFR 20.1502	Conditions requiring individual monitoring of external and internal occupational dose.
10 CFR 20.1701	Use of process or other engineering controls.
10 CFR 20.1702	Use of other controls.

The complete text of these regulations can be accessed online through the NRC electronic reading room at www.nrc.gov.

For those individuals assigned to work environments in which inhalation or ingestion of radioactive material is possible, derived air concentration (DAC) and annual limit on intake (ALI) values, provided by the NRC in Table 1 of Appendix B to Part 20, may be used to determine occupational dose.

10 CFR 20.1202 Compliance with requirements for summation of external and internal doses.

If a licensee is required to monitor workers for both external and internal radiation dose under § 20.1502, the licensee must demonstrate compliance with the annual occupational dose limits by summing both contributions.

10 CFR 20.1203 Determination of external dose from airborne radioactive material.

The external dose, for situations in which an individual is working in an area where airborne radioactive materials exist, should be based on measurements using individual monitoring devices or survey instruments.

10 CFR 20.1204 Determination of internal exposure.

If a licensee is required to measure internal dose under § 20.1502 to demonstrate compliance with occupational dose limits, the licensee must take suitable and timely measurements of:

(1) Concentrations of radioactive materials in air in work areas;

(2) Quantities of radionuclides in the body;

(3) Quantities of radionuclides excreted from the body; or

(4) Combinations of these measurements

Unless respiratory protective equipment is used or the assessment of intake is based on bioassays, the licensee must assume that an individual inhales the airborne concentration present.

10 CFR 20.1207 Occupational dose limits for minors.

Annual occupational dose limits for minors (individuals under the age of 18 y) are 10% of those specified for adult workers.

10 CFR 20.1208 Dose to an embryo/fetus.

The dose equivalent to an embryo/fetus in occupational exposure of a declared pregnant woman, must not exceed 0.5 rem (5 mSv) during an entire pregnancy. Efforts must be made to maintain a uniform monthly exposure rate.

If dose to embryo/fetus has reached or exceeded 0.45 rem (4.5 mSv) by the time the woman declares her pregnancy to the licensee, the embryo/fetus may receive an additional 0.05 rem (0.5 mSv) during the remainder of the pregnancy and still be in compliance.

10 CFR 20.1501 General.

All personnel dosimeters that require processing to determine the radiation dose and that are used by licensees to comply with § 20.1201 must be processed and evaluated by an approved and accredited dosimetry processor (accreditation from the National Voluntary Laboratory Accreditation Program [NVLAP] of the National Institute of Standards and Technology).

10 CFR 20.1502 Conditions requiring individual monitoring of external and internal occupational dose.

Exposures to radiation and radioactive material must be monitored at levels sufficient to demonstrate compliance with the occupational dose limits.

Diagnostic nuclear medicine licensees must monitor the occupational external exposure and must supply and require the use of individual monitoring devices by all of the following individuals:

(1) Adults likely to receive an annual external dose >10% of the limits in § 20.1201(a) (e.g., 0.5 rem [5 mSv]);

(2) Minors likely to receive an annual external dose >0.1 rem (1 mSv), an LDE >0.15 rem (1.5 mSv), or an SDE >0.5 rem (5 mSv); and

(3) Declared pregnant women likely to receive an external dose >0.1 rem (1 mSv) during an entire pregnancy.

Diagnostic nuclear medicine licensees must also monitor the occupational intake of radioactive material and assess the committed effective dose equivalent (CEDE) to all of the following individuals:

(1) Adults likely to receive an annual intake >10% of the applicable annual limit on intake (ALI);

(2) Minors likely to receive an annual CEDE >0.1 rem (1 mSv); and

(3) Declared pregnant women likely to receive a CEDE >0.1 rem (1 mSv) during an entire pregnancy.

10 CFR 20.1701 Use of process or other engineering controls.

The licensee must use, to the extent practical, process or other engineering controls (e.g., containment or ventilation) to control the concentrations of radioactive material in air.

10 CFR 20.1702 Use of other controls.

When it is not practical to apply process or other engineering controls to control the concentrations of radioactive material in air to values below those that define an airborne radioactivity area, the licensee must, consistent with maintaining the total effective dose equivalent as low as reasonably achievable (ALARA), increase monitoring and limit intakes by one or more of the following means: control of access, limitation of exposure times, use of respiratory protection equipment, or other controls.

9.2.2 Discussion of the Requirements

The licensee, to the extent practical, must achieve occupational doses that are not only within regulatory limits but also ALARA. Licensees must either:

(1) Monitor external and/or internal occupational radiation exposure; or

(2) Demonstrate that an unmonitored individual is not likely to receive a radiation dose >10% of the occupational dose limits.

In the latter case, vigilance should be maintained to ensure that current programs continue to meet regulatory requirements. Even if licensees are not required to monitor employees, they still may choose to do so.

Radiation workers potentially can receive radiation doses in two distinct ways: external exposure and internal intake. The TEDE concept makes it possible to combine these dose components in assessing the overall risk to the health of an individual. The TEDE is equal to the sum of the DDE, resulting from external exposures, and the CEDE, resulting from internal exposures. These two sources of radiation dose also must be considered for demonstrating compliance with the annual dose limit for any individual organ or tissue, known as the total organ dose equivalent (TODE). In this case, CEDE is replaced by the committed dose equivalent (CDE). The relationship among these values is expressed as:

$$\mathbf{TODE = CDE + DDE.} \qquad (9\text{-}1)$$

Licensees often decide to monitor all workers who are likely to be exposed to radioactive materials, regardless of the magnitude of the exposure. However, personnel monitoring devices for measurement of external dose are required for only those workers likely to receive exposures in excess of the specified threshold of 500 mrem (5 mSv) from external radiation sources. Likewise, licensees are also required to monitor only the occupational intakes of those workers who are likely to exceed 10% of the specific ALI or CEDE limit. An intake of activity can occur by ingestion, inhalation, or skin absorption. The likelihood of internal intake by ingestion or inhalation depends on the radionuclide and the attached agent (e.g., for ^{99m}Tc-labeled radiopharmaceuticals, the likely route, probably quite minimal, would be ingestion).

9.2.2.1 Internal Component of Occupational Radiation Dose

If it can be demonstrated by air sampling or calculations that adult radiation workers are not likely to receive an annual intake >10% of an ALI (i.e., a CEDE per year dose of 500 mrem [5 mSv]), because the intake of 1 ALI results in a CEDE of 5 rem (0.05 Sv) and

TABLE 9.2

Dose Conversion Factors and Resulting CEDEs for Commonly Used Radionuclides

Radionuclide (Activity [mCi])	Ingestion DCF (rem/mCi*) (CEDE [mrem])		Inhalation DCF (rem/mCi) (CEDE [mrem])	
^{18}F (10)	0.12	(0.012)	0.08	(0.008)
^{67}Ga (5)	0.78	(0.039)	0.35	(0.018)
^{99m}Tc (20)	0.06	(0.012)	0.03	(0.006)
^{111}In (0.5)	1.32	(0.0066)	0.77	(0.0039)
^{123}I (10)	0.53	(0.053)	0.30	(0.03)
^{131}I (0.03)	53.28	(0.016)	32.89	(0.0099)
^{133}Xe (15)	—		—	
^{201}Tl (2)	0.30	(0.006)	0.23	(0.0046)

*SI conversion: 1 rem = 0.01 Sv; 1 mCi = 37 MBq.

DCF = dose conversion factor; CEDE = committed effective dose equivalent.

that minors and declared pregnant women are not likely to receive a CEDE >100 mrem (1 mSv) (i.e., 2% of an ALI), then monitoring occupational intakes in these individuals would not be required. Appendix B to Part 20 specifies ALIs (in microcuries) of radionuclides for occupational exposure. The ALIs in the appendix are the annual intakes of a given radionuclide that would result in either: (1) a CEDE of 5 rem (0.05 Sv) (stochastic ALI); or (2) a CEDE of 50 rem (0.5 Sv) to an organ or tissue (nonstochastic ALI). However, these ALIs are based on generalized metabolic and biochemical properties and are not recommended for use by diagnostic nuclear medicine licensees. When specific information on the physical and biochemical properties of the radionuclides taken into the body or the behavior of the material in an individual is known, the licensee may use that information to calculate the CEDE (§ 20.1204 (c)).

According to NUREG-1556, Vol. 9, Appendix U, *Release of Patients Administered Radioactive Materials,* an estimate of the maximum likely internal dose (i.e., CEDE) to an individual exposed to a radioactivity source (in rem) from internal exposure can be calculated as:

$$\mathbf{CEDE = Q \times 10^{-5} \times DCF,} \qquad (9\text{-}2)$$

where Q = activity handled (mCi), 10^{-5} = assumed fractional intake, and DCF = dose conversion factor (rem/mCi).

A common rule of thumb or heuristic is to assume that no more than 1 millionth of the activity being handled will become an intake to an individual working with radioactive material. This rule was developed for cases of worker intakes during normal workplace operations and from accidental exposures and public intakes from accidental airborne releases from a facility. The value of 10^{-5} was chosen to add a degree of conservatism to the calculation. The DCF converts intakes in millicuries to an internal CEDE, and values are available for both the ingestion and inhalation pathway in Federal Guidance Report No. 11, *Limiting Values of Radionuclide Intake and Air Concentration and Dose Conversion Factors for Inhalation, Submersion, and Ingestion.* These values and the resulting CEDEs for the most commonly used radionuclides in diagnostic nuclear medicine are shown in Table 9.2.

All values of the CEDE are extremely low and demonstrate that the dose component resulting from internal intake is not likely to pose any danger for individuals as a result of diagnostic nuclear medicine procedures. For example, the highest estimated CEDE (0.03 mrem [0.3 μSv]) resulting from inhalation is associated with the use of 10 mCi (370 MBq) ^{123}I. For an adult worker to exceed the 10%-of-the-ALI threshold (i.e., a 500-mrem [5 mSv] CEDE) and trigger the requirement for occupational intake monitoring, that individual would have to perform more than 65 of these procedures per day (a minor or declared pregnant woman would have to perform more than 13 procedures per day to exceed the 100 mrem [1 mSv] CEDE threshold)—an unlikely possibility. Thus, diagnostic nuclear medicine licensees are not required to monitor the internal component of the occupational radiation dose. Note that CEDEs were not calculated for ^{133}Xe, the radioactive gas most likely to be used in diagnostic nuclear medicine, because it poses no internal hazard. If an individual is working in an area in which airborne ^{133}Xe might be present, the preferred method of determining worker exposure is by radiation dose measurements using personnel dosimeters to record the DDE, a measure of external dose.

It is important to note that, because of differences in biodistribution, the DCFs used to generate Table 9.2 are accurate for the radionuclide but not necessarily for the radiopharmaceutical from which the intake may occur. In any case, intakes from the radionuclide with the greatest potential for intake (i.e., ^{131}I) have been monitored for years without any significant occurrences. Therefore, the likelihood of a worker receiving an intake of any other nonvolatile radionuclide used in diagnostic nuclear medicine that would exceed the regulatory limit is exceedingly small and is additional support for not performing internal dose monitoring.

Almost all diagnostic nuclear medicine licensees, then, can demonstrate compliance with the annual dose limits by monitoring only external exposure. Three annual occupational dose limits apply to external exposure:

(1) DDE to the whole body (5 rem [0.05 Sv] for the case of no internal intake);

(2) LDE to the lens of the eye (15 rem [0.15 Sv]); and

(3) SDE to the skin or extremities (50 rem [0.50 Sv]).

If protective lenses are worn, it is acceptable to take the shielding into account when evaluating the LDE. Monitoring an individual's external radiation exposure is required if the external occupational dose is likely to exceed 10% of the appropriate dose limit:

(1) For adults likely to receive an annual dose >0.5 rem (5 mSv) DDE, >1.5 rem (15 mSv) LDE, or >5 rem (0.05 Sv) SDE;

(2) For minors likely to receive an annual dose >0.1 rem (1 mSv) DDE, >0.15 rem (1.5 mSv) LDE, or >0.5 rem (5 mSv) SDE; and

(3) For declared pregnant women likely to receive >0.1 rem (1 mSv) DDE during the entire pregnancy. The licensee must make efforts to avoid substantial variation above a uniform monthly exposure rate.

Each licensee must advise each worker annually of the worker's dose as contained in records maintained by the licensee. If it can be demonstrated that workers are not likely to exceed 10% of the annual occupational external dose limits, they are not required to be monitored. Prior experience is the best method to demonstrate worker dose levels; that is, licensees should review their historical occupational radiation doses to determine whether workers are likely to receive external doses >10% of the limits.

9.2.2.2 External Component of Occupational Radiation Dose

Personnel dosimeters (e.g., film badges, thermoluminescent dosimeters [TLDs], and optically stimulated luminescent dosimeters [OSLs]) measure doses received by only a small portion of the body. For monitoring purposes, the doses recorded must reflect the highest dose received; that is, the dosimeter must be representative of the maximum dose. Licensees should ensure that their personnel dosimetry program contains provisions that personnel monitoring devices be worn so that the part of the body likely to receive the greatest dose will be monitored. If occupational workers handle (e.g., prepare or inject) licensed material and are likely to receive a dose >5 rem (0.05 Sv) SDE, the licensee should evaluate the need to provide extremity dosimeters (e.g., ring badges).

The SDE refers to two distinct areas of the body: the skin of the whole body and the skin of the extremities. The dose limits apply to any specified region of the skin or extremities, and the doses to different regions are not additive (i.e., the doses to different regions should be tracked separately). Radioactive material on the skin can result in a radiation dose to the skin that can be evaluated with available software, such as VARSKIN Mod 2 (Pacific Northwest Laboratory, Richland, WA). Likewise, if a licensee's program involves the potential for significant doses to the lens of the eye, additional evaluations must be performed to assess those doses.

One additional note is relevant for licensees using radioactive gases or aerosols (e.g., ^{133}Xe or ^{81m}Kr gas and ^{99m}Tc aerosols) for lung scintigraphy. As noted previously, the diagnostic nuclear medicine licensee is not required to monitor the internal component of the occupational radiation dose of workers with these radionuclides. However, pursuant to § 20.1701, the licensee must use process or other engineering controls (e.g., containment, decontamination, or ventilation) to the extent practical to control the concentrations of radioactive material in the air. Radioactive contamination of the air can occur as a result of the use of radioactive gases but is unlikely with aerosols (e.g., ^{99m}Tc-diethylenetriaminepentaacetic acid is administered through a nebulizer that creates a fine mist of radioactive particles that, if released into the room, will settle to the floor). This level of airborne radioactive material must be below the DAC value for the specific radionuclide. The DAC is the value of the air concentration of a specific radionuclide in microcuries per milliliter, which, if breathed continuously for a working year of 40 h/wk for 50 weeks (2,000 hours total), would result in an intake of 1 ALI or a CEDE of 5 rem (0.05 Sv). One DAC, if breathed continuously for 1 hour (1 DAC-h), would result in a CEDE of 2.5 mrem (0.025 mSv). Because the DAC is intended to control chronic occupational exposures, it represents a time-averaged value and not an instantaneous value. Thus, airborne concentrations at any given time may be above the DAC value. For gases such as ^{133}Xe, the DAC is calculated directly from the external dose. Therefore, dose calculations involving the restricted area DAC of 1×10^{-4} µCi/mL for ^{133}Xe represent a DDE.

As an example, consider the release of 2 mCi (74 MBq) ^{133}Xe (20% of a typical administered activity of 10 mCi [370 MBq]) in an unventilated room that measures 12 × 12 × 8 feet (1,152 cubic feet [cft]). The instantaneous airborne radioactivity concentration in this room would initially be quite large and then decrease rapidly as the gas fills the entire room. At that time, the radioactivity concentration in the room air could be expressed as:

$$C = A/V, \tag{9-3}$$

where C is the airborne radioactivity concentration in the room in microcuries per milliliter, A is the activity in microcuries released into the room, and V is the volume of the room in milliliters. (A useful volume conversion factor is 1 cft ≅ 28,300 mL). Thus:

$$C\,(\mu Ci/mL) = 2000\,\mu Ci/(1{,}152\text{ cft} \times 28{,}300\text{ mL/cft}) = 6 \times 10^{-5}\,\mu Ci/mL, \tag{9-4}$$

a value lower than the DAC limit. However, if multiple studies are performed in this room every week throughout the year, the airborne radioactivity concentration in the room would be higher and, in this case, might exceed the DAC limit. Consideration should also be given to the likelihood of leakage into surrounding unrestricted areas.

Therefore, to more rapidly eliminate airborne activity concentrations of gases during normal operations or in the event of accidental gas "spills," the room may have to be adequately ventilated so that contaminated air is exchanged and diluted with noncontaminated air. Adequate ventilation of room air can be accomplished by either direct venting to the atmosphere through an air exhaust system (the room should be under negative pressure to ensure that the exhaust is vented and not recirculated or allowed to migrate into the surrounding unrestricted areas) or by collecting airborne radioactivity in a shielded container (e.g., xenon or aerosol traps) for subsequent decay and disposal. The choice should be based on the effluent air concentration that may be released to the environment (see section 9.3). Because worker exposure to ^{133}Xe gas is best documented by personnel dosimeter readings, licensees can use their historical occupational dosimetry data to assess the need for room ventilation as part of their ALARA programs.

The previous example of ^{133}Xe gas release can be used to illustrate how room ventilation works. The unventilated room measuring 12 × 12 × 8 feet is now directly vented to the outside atmosphere. The airborne radioactivity concentration in the room, as a function of time, can be expressed as:

$$C = (A/V) \times e^{-tQ/V}, \tag{9-5}$$

where C is the airborne radioactivity concentration in the room in microcuries per minute at time t, A is the activity in microcuries released into the room, V is the volume of the room in milliliters; t is the time in minutes; and Q is the exhaust rate in milliliters per minute. Note that Q/V in the exponential term represents the air

TABLE 9.3

Room Air Concentration (µCi/mL)

Time	Room air changes per minute			
(min)	0.01	0.1	0.5	1
0	A/V	A/V	A/V	A/V
1	0.99 x A/V	0.90 x A/V	0.61 x A/V	0.37 x A/V
5	0.95 x A/V	0.61 x A/V	0.08 x A/V	0.01 x A/V
10	0.90 x A/V	0.37 x A/V	0.01 x A/V	0.00005 x A/V

A = activity in microcuries released into room; V = volume of room in milliliters.

exchange rate or the number of times that the ventilation system replaces the air in the room (e.g., for our room of 1,152 cft, an air exhaust rate of 115.2 cft/min would result in 0.1 room air changes/min). Assuming that the initial air radioactivity concentration at time 0 is equal to A/V, Table 9.3 illustrates how quickly this initial concentration would be reduced.

Obviously, the greater the room exhaust rate, the faster the room radioactivity concentration decreases. Based on these exhaust rates, the average air concentration of radioactivity in the room can also be estimated easily, because:

$$\text{C } (\mu\text{Ci/mL}) = \text{total activity released } (\mu\text{Ci})/\text{total exhausted air volume (mL)} = A/(Q \times t), \quad (9\text{-}6)$$

where A is the total activity released per week (equal to 2×10^4 μCi [740 MBq], assuming 10 patients per week and that an average of 2 mCi [74 MBq] ^{133}Xe are released into the room per study), Q is the air exhaust rate in milliliters per minute, and t is the length of the work week (40 h/wk × 60 min/h = 2,400 min), assuming that the ventilation system operates continuously during this time. If only a few studies are performed on a weekly basis, it may be prudent to have the system on only during the procedure, if possible. Note that Q × t is the total exhausted air volume in milliliters. For our example room size, the air exchange rates per minute of 0.01, 0.1, 0.5, and 1 correspond to 11.52, 115.2, 576, and 1,152 cft/min (cfm), respectively. The result for 11.52 cfm is:

$$\text{C } (\mu\text{Ci/mL}) = 2 \times 10^4\ \mu\text{Ci})/[(11.52\text{ cfm})(28{,}300\text{ mL/cft})(2{,}400\text{ min})] = 2.6 \times 10^{-5}\ \mu\text{Ci/mL}, \quad (9\text{-}7)$$

for 115.2 cfm:

$$\text{C } (\mu\text{Ci/mL}) = 2.6 \times 10^{-6}\ \mu\text{Ci/mL}; \quad (9\text{-}8)$$

for 576 cfm:

$$\text{C } (\mu\text{Ci/mL}) = 5.1 \times 10^{-7}\ \mu\text{Ci/mL}; \text{ and} \quad (9\text{-}9)$$

for 1,152 cfm:

$$\text{C } (\mu\text{Ci/mL}) = 2.6 \times 10^{-7}\ \mu\text{Ci/mL}. \quad (9\text{-}10)$$

All values of room air concentration are well below the DAC limit for a restricted area. Using an exhaust rate of 115.2 cfm, a worker continuously exposed to ^{133}Xe in an air concentration of 2.6×10^{-6} μCi/mL is likely to receive an external dose (i.e., DDE) of 130 mrem, which is <10% of the applicable dose limit.

It would be reasonable to ask what exhaust rate would be sufficient to maintain the air concentration of radioactivity below the regulatory limit. In this case, we want to limit C to 1×10^{-4} μCi/mL (the restricted area DAC for ^{133}Xe). The required minimum room exhaust rate for our example room can be expressed as:

$$Q = A/(C \times 2{,}400) = 2 \times 10^4\ \mu\text{Ci}/\ [(1 \times 10^{-4}\ \mu\text{Ci/mL})(2{,}400\text{ min})] = 83{,}000\text{ mL/min} = 2.9\text{ cfm}. \quad (9\text{-}11)$$

It should be noted that procedures necessary to determine the appropriate room exhaust rate may vary considerably. A minimum air flow that results in a number of air exchanges and complies with requirements of the Uniform Mechanical Code can be used, although this will usually result in air flows in excess of NRC requirements and will consequently waste energy and money. Instead, calculations can be performed to determine the minimum air flow necessary. If the licensee decides to simply ensure that the room is under negative pressure (the requirement that the room be under negative pressure has been removed from the regulations), no air flow calculations need be performed. In addition, it should be determined whether the ventilation system should be operated continuously (e.g., if many studies are performed) or turned on only occasionally (e.g., if few studies are performed). Then, using the room air exhaust rate, calculations taking into account the licensee's facility and workload, as specified previously, can be used to demonstrate compliance in controlling the concentrations of radioactive gas in the room air.

9.2.3 Suggested Procedures for Compliance

Based on the principles of radiation protection, diagnostic nuclear medicine licensees must develop policies and procedures to minimize radiation dose to workers from both external exposure and internal contamination. It is necessary to assess doses to radiation workers to demonstrate compliance with regulatory limits on radiation dose and to help demonstrate that doses are maintained at ALARA levels. Exposure of nuclear medicine personnel to radiation can occur from three main activities: dosage preparation and assay, injection, and patient imaging.

9.2.3.1 Model Procedure for Monitoring External Dose

External radiation exposure (including radiation exposure to hands and fingers of individuals involved in injecting dosages or handling radioactive materials in the hot lab) is controlled by the classic methods of time, distance, and shielding. Syringe shields are effective and are used in kit preparation of radiopharmaceuticals and during patient administration, if possible. Shielding in hot labs is provided, as necessary, as well as tongs to further minimize worker exposure.

External dose is determined by using individual monitoring devices (e.g., film badges, TLDs, or OSLs). These devices are evaluated by a dosimetry processor that is NVLAP-approved. Acceptable exchange frequencies are every month for film badges and every 3 months for TLDs and OSLs. These badges may be processed on a monthly basis to more rapidly assess dose trends.

The device for monitoring the whole-body, eye, skin, or extremity dose will be placed near the location expected to receive the highest dose during the year. When the whole body is exposed fairly uniformly, the monitoring device typically will be worn on the front of the upper torso. If the radiation dose is nonuniform, so that a specific part of the whole body receives a substantially higher dose than the rest of the body (e.g., as occurs in handling radioactive material), the monitoring device is placed near that part of the body. Typically, ring dosimeters are worn in addition to whole-body dosimeters by the individuals (e.g., technologists) who handle the radioactive material.

It is important that licensees ensure that users return personnel monitoring devices on time and get a new device each time one is turned in for processing. Licensees must also do all they can to recover missing devices. If an individual's device is lost, the licensee should perform and document an evaluation of the dose the individual received during that period and add it to the worker's dose record. Sometimes the most reliable method for estimating this dose is to use the worker's recent dose history. In other cases, it may be better to use doses of co-workers as a basis for the dose estimate.

For declared pregnant workers, procedures with potentially higher exposures might be discontinued, if possible. If these procedures are performed, adequate shielding should be considered and the worker should be extremely conscientious in avoiding personal contamination. For example, a lead apron or half-apron may be worn. A fetal dosimeter is worn under the apron on the abdominal region, and a whole-body dosimeter is worn over the apron so that the dose to the fetus and the dose to the worker may be monitored independently. To take advantage of the lower exposure limit (i.e., 0.5 rem [5 mSv]) and the associated dose monitoring provisions, a woman must declare her pregnancy in writing to the licensee. Such a declaration derives from legal, not health, considerations. It is important to state that a woman's decision to declare her pregnancy is entirely voluntary. A declared pregnant woman also has the right to "undeclare" her pregnancy. In such an event, the licensee will withdraw any restrictive measures or enhanced monitoring established to comply with the embryo/fetus dose limits. It is also important to remember that any information about a worker's pregnancy is confidential.

Personnel monitoring results are recorded on NRC Form 5, which can be obtained at the NRC's Web site (www.nrc.gov/reading-rm/doc-collections/forms/), or an equivalent form (e.g., dosimetry processor's report). The licensee must advise each worker required to be monitored of their dose on an annual basis, pursuant to § 20.1502. The licensee must also review results of personnel monitoring in the context of ALARA practices. If dose histories indicate that workers receive >10% of the applicable dose limits, these workers will continue to be monitored. For those workers who receive doses that approach the annual limits and are not consistent with good ALARA practices, the licensee should investigate work habits and determine whether any potential additional safety measures are needed to reduce worker dose.

Licensees will use this review as an opportunity to determine whether these radiation dose histories

Regulatory Issues at a Glance: Occupational Dose Limits

- Dose limits for adults
- Dose limits for minors
- Declared pregnant workers
- Dose limits for embryo/fetus
- External dose
- Internal dose
- Summation of external and internal dose
- Monitoring devices
- Airborne radioactive materials
- Notifications and reports to workers

might permit the reduction in or elimination of the need for monitoring workers. Workers who consistently receive <10% of the applicable dose limits may no longer need to be monitored for radiation doses. These data also will be used to determine if the nature and frequency of the required radiation surveys (see section 9.6) can be further reduced. Before any changes are made to the radiation protection program based on this review, they will be reviewed and approved by the radiation safety officer and licensee management, and all affected individuals will be instructed on the revised program (§ 35.26).

For rooms in which radioactive gases or aerosols are employed, appropriate ventilation must be considered, depending on the size of the room and the number of studies performed on a weekly basis. (Licensees may refer to the examples given here and use them as a guide for their own facility design and operating procedures.) Established licensees also should base their continued need for room ventilation on historical dosimetry data. In addition, all xenon containers, both pre- and postadministration, are shielded and stored in a well-ventilated fume hood. Nebulizers containing ^{99m}Tc are also shielded, and care is taken to assemble the nebulizer according to the manufacturer's instructions. If necessary, absorbent paper should be placed to minimize the spread of radioactive contamination and facilitate decontamination when nebulizers are used.

9.2.3.2 Model Procedure for Monitoring Internal Dose (None Required)

The types and quantities of radioactive material manipulated at almost all diagnostic nuclear medicine facilities do not provide a reasonable possibility for internal intake by workers. All values of the CEDE resulting from ingestion and inhalation of commonly used radionuclides in diagnostic nuclear medicine have been shown to be extremely low and further demonstrate that the dose component from internal intake is not likely to pose any danger for individuals. Thus, diagnostic nuclear medicine licensees usually are not required to monitor the internal component of the radiation dose, and the TEDE is given simply by the DDE from external exposure.

9.3 Dose Limits for Members of the Public

9.3.1 Pertinent Regulations

10 CFR 20.1101 Radiation protection programs.

There must be a constraint on air emissions of radioactive material to the environment such that a member of the public is not expected to receive a total effective dose equivalent (TEDE) in excess of 10 mrem (0.1 mSv) per year.

10 CFR 20.1301 Dose limits for individual members of the public.

Each licensee must conduct operations so that:

(1) The annual TEDE to individual members of the public does not exceed 0.1 rem (1 mSv); this dose limit is exclusive of dose contribu-

Dose Limits for Members of the Public

Pertinent regulations:

10 CFR 20.1101	Radiation protection programs.
10 CFR 20.1301	Dose limits for individual members of the public.
10 CFR 20.1302	Compliance with dose limits for individual members of the public.
10 CFR 35.75	Release of individuals containing unsealed byproduct material or implants containing byproduct material.

The complete text of these regulations can be accessed online through the NRC electronic reading room at www.nrc.gov.

tions from background radiation, from any medical administration the individual has received, from exposure to individuals administered radioactive materials and released in accordance with § 35.75, from voluntary participation in medical research programs, and from the licensee's disposal of radioactive material into sanitary sewerage; and

(2) The dose in any unrestricted area from external sources (exclusive of dose contributions from patients released in accordance with § 35.75) does not exceed 2 mrem (0.02 mSv) in any 1 hour.

10 CFR 20.1302 Compliance with dose limits for individual members of the public.

Licensees must make, as appropriate, surveys of radiation levels in unrestricted and controlled areas to demonstrate compliance with the dose limits for individual members of the public in § 20.1301.

Licensees must show compliance with the annual public dose limit. One way to do this is by demonstrating by measurement or calculation that the TEDE to the individual likely to receive the highest dose does not exceed this limit.

10 CFR 35.75 Release of individuals containing unsealed byproduct material or implants containing byproduct material.

Licensees must provide instructions to a lactating individual who has been administered unsealed byproduct material if the total effective dose equivalent to a nursing infant or child could exceed 0.1 rem (1 mSv) assuming there were no interruption of breast feeding. These instructions must include guidance on the interruption or discontinuation of breast feeding and information on the potential consequences, if any, of failure to follow the guidance.

9.3.2 Discussion of the Requirements

The dose to the public is controlled by ensuring that licensed material is used, transported, and stored in such a way that members of the public will not receive >100 mrem (1 mSv) in 1 year and that the dose in any unrestricted area is not >2 mrem (0.02 mSv) in any 1 hour. To properly control public dose, licensed material must be secured to prevent unauthorized access or use by individuals coming into the area. Many sources of exposure are excluded from the public dose limits, and licensees may seek NRC approval to increase the annual public dose limit. The dose limit of 2 mrem (0.02 mSv) in any 1 hour is not a dose rate but a dose in a period of time. This allows for instantaneous dose rates in unrestricted areas to be >2 mrem/h (0.02 mSv/h) as long as these dose rates remain <2 mrem when averaged over an hour. For example, an instantaneous dose rate of 120 mrem/h (1.2 mSv/h) may exist for 1 minute, provided that the dose rate does not exceed background for the remaining 59 minutes.

For the annual cumulative dose limit, the licensee must make an effort to determine which individual is likely to receive the highest exposure (i.e., the individual closest to restricted areas or most likely to frequent these areas). In many cases, this individual is the facility's receptionist or secretary. A reasonable estimate of the external radiation dose to the member of the public likely to receive the highest dose can be calculated using the following scenario. Assume that this individual is a receptionist or secretary who is considered a member of the public, spends 1,750 hours/year in the facility (7 h/day for 50 wk/y), and works at a desk in an unrestricted area at a conservative distance of 5 meters from the facility's restricted areas. To exceed the annual public dose limit of 100 mrem (1 mSv), 6.5 mCi (240.5 MBq) ^{131}I, 19 mCi (703 MBq) ^{67}Ga, or 19 mCi (703 MBq) ^{99m}Tc would have to be continuously irradiating this individual (assuming that no shielding of any kind was involved). In each case, the dose rate in any 1 hour would be equal to 0.057 mrem (0.57 μSv), less than the 2 - mrem (0.02 mSv) limit.

This conservative scenario demonstrates that it is improbable that any member of the public at a diagnostic medical facility will receive an annual radiation dose or dose rate in 1 hour that exceeds applicable dose limits. As previously noted, the dose limit in any 1 hour as defined is exclusive of dose contributions from radioactive patients and pertains only to dose contributions from radioactive materials (e.g., in syringes, in sealed sources, or on the floor after a contamination incident).

The dose limit constraint of 10 mrem/year (0.1 mSv/y) is an as-low-as-reasonably-achievable requirement and applies only to the release of airborne radioactive effluents to the environment. This dose limit would be satisfied if it can be demonstrated that no individual is likely to be exposed to >10% of the appropriate derived air concentration (DAC) provided by the NRC in Appendix B to Part 20 (Table 2) for the potential offending radionuclide. The DAC limit for ^{133}Xe, for example, for unrestricted areas is 5×10^{-7} μCi/mL. This represents the air concentration that would result in an external dose of 100 mrem (1 mSv) to a member of the public exposed continuously (i.e., 24 h/day all year). (The 100-mrem dose applies to those DAC values for radionuclides that pose only an external hazard; for all other radionuclides, the DAC limits if inhaled or ingested continuously over the course of a year would produce a TEDE of 50 mrem [0.5 mSv].) In this case, 10 mrem/year (0.1 mSv/y) would result if an individual were continuously exposed to >20% of the appropriate DAC. It is highly unlikely that any member of the public would be exposed continuously to such an activity concentration.

An example is the room used for ^{133}Xe imaging studies described in section 9.2. The room has a continuously operating ventilation system with an exhaust rate of 115.2 cft/min ≅ 1 cft × 28,300 mL), and the average number of ^{133}Xe studies per week is 10, each involving a release of 2 mCi (74 MBq) ^{133}Xe (20% of the average administered activity of 10 mCi (370 MBq) into the room. In this case, the total estimated release of activity per year can be expressed as:

$$\mathbf{10\ patients/wk \times 52\ wk/y \times 2\ mCi/patient = 1 \times 10^{6}\ \mu Ci/year.} \quad (9\text{-}12)$$

The total air volume released per year is:

$$\mathbf{115.2\ cft/min \times 28{,}300\ mL/cft \times 5.26 \times 10^{5}\ min/y = 1.7 \times 10^{12}\ mL/y,} \quad (9\text{-}13)$$

and the average yearly concentration (C) is equal to:

$$C = \frac{1 \times 10^{6}\ \mu Ci/y}{1.7 \times 10^{12}\ mL/y} = 6 \times 10^{-7}\ \mu Ci/mL. \quad (9\text{-}14)$$

Because, in our example of ^{133}Xe, C is approximately 10 times larger than 10% of the unrestricted area DAC of 0.5×10^{-7} μCi/mL, it might be assumed that licensees must increase the exhaust rate of the room by a factor of 10 or use xenon or aerosol traps. However, as calculated, the air concentration is extremely conservative. It assumes that 20% of every administration will result in air contamination, and it represents the value at the exhaust location of the ventilation system. The air concentration of radioactivity will be significantly lower at other locations because of dilution. In addition, if the exhaust vent is appropriately placed, it would be unreasonable to assume that a member of the public would be at this location continuously, if at all. Thus, this limited occupancy factor (certainly <0.1) and atmospheric dilution factor would most likely bring the air emissions rate of radioactive material into compliance with the regulations. If we assume an extremely conservative occupancy factor of 0.04 (i.e., 1 h/day), C would equal 0.2×10^{-7} μCi/mL, which is below the DAC limit. Each licensee must demonstrate in its facility design and/or its use of other controls that the TEDE (essentially the deep-dose equivalent) to that member of the public most likely to receive the highest dose from airborne releases to the environment is not expected to exceed the regulatory limit. Thus, the exhaust rate for rooms in which radioactive gases and aerosols are used and, more important, the location of the exhaust vent (see also section 9.4) should be such that a member of the public is not expected to receive a TEDE >10 mrem/y (0.1 mSv/y).

If a lactating individual has been administered unsealed byproduct material and the TEDE to a nursing infant or child could exceed 0.1 rem (1mSv) assuming there were no interruption of breast feeding, instructions must be provided. These instructions must include guidance on the interruption or disontinuation of breast feeding and information on the potential consequences, if any, of failure to follow the guidance. As discussed in Chapter 2, a dose >0.1 rem is highly unlikely as a result of most diagnostic nuclear medicine procedures.

9.3.3 Suggested Procedures for Compliance

The licensee must control and maintain constant surveillance of licensed material that is not in storage, as well as secure stored licensed material in a locked room to prevent unauthorized access, removal, or use.

> **Regulatory Issues at a Glance**
> **Dose Limits for Members of the Public**
>
> Dose limits for the public maintained
> Air emissions to environment
> Radiation surveys
> Lactating patient and breast feeding infant.

Licensed material must be located so that the public dose in an unrestricted area does not exceed 100 mrem (1 mSv) in 1 year or 2 mrem (0.02 mSv) in any 1 hour. The licensee must comply with both these limits and use concepts of time, distance, and shielding when choosing storage and use locations. Occasional surveys of radiation levels in unrestricted areas should be performed (see section 9.6). (A calculation was presented in 9.3.2 to ensure that the public dose limit was maintained based on the exposure rate constants for three unshielded radionuclides at a given distance from an employee's office. Licensees should redo the calculation based on their facility layout and the radionuclides used most often.)

There is a constraint on air emissions of radioactive material to the environment so that a member of the public is not expected to receive a TEDE >10 mrem/y (0.1 mSv/y). (A calculation was presented in 9.3.2. Each licensee should redo the calculation to demonstrate compliance with this dose limit based on their facility layout and operating procedures).

If a lactating woman undergoes a diagnostic nuclear medicine procedure and it is likely that a breast feeding infant or child could receive a radiation dose that will exceed 0.1 rem (mSv), the licensee must instruct the patient about breast feeding options (interruption or cessation) and the potential consequences, if any, of failure to follow these instructions.

9.4 Minimization of Contamination/Spill Procedures

9.4.1 Pertinent Regulations

10 CFR 20.1406 Minimization of contamination.
Applicants for licenses, other than renewals, must describe in the application how facility design and procedures for operation will minimize, to the extent practicable, contamination of the facility and the environment, facilitate eventual decommissioning, and minimize, to the extent practicable, the generation of radioactive waste.

10 CFR 30.35 Financial assurance and recordkeeping for decommissioning.
Each licensee must keep records of information (e.g., spills) important to the decommissioning of a facility in an identified location until the site is released for unrestricted use. These records may be limited to instances when contamination remains after any cleanup procedures.

Minimization of Contamination/Spill Procedures

Pertinent regulations:

10 CFR 20.1406	Minimization of contamination.
10 CFR 30.35	Financial assurance and recordkeeping for decommissioning.

The complete text of these regulations can be accessed online through the NRC electronic reading room at www.nrc.gov.

9.4.2 Discussion of the Requirements

Applicants are required to submit a facility diagram in the license application (see section 10.1). When designing facilities and developing procedures for the safe use of licensed materials, new applicants should consider how to minimize radioactive contamination and the generation of radioactive waste. The facilities (and equipment) must be adequate to protect health and minimize danger to life or property (§ 30.33(a)(2)). To achieve this goal, new applicants should:

(1) Implement and adhere to good health physics practices;
(2) Minimize areas in which licensed materials will be used and stored;
(3) Establish frequency and scope of radiation surveys;
(4) Determine whether filtration is necessary in effluent streams;
(5) Use nonporous materials in radioactive material use and storage areas; and
(6) Employ ventilation stacks and ductwork with minimal lengths and minimal abrupt changes in direction so that they exhaust into the environment in a location not likely to result in an appreciable exposure to any individual.

This regulation is intended to minimize the potential impact of radioactive contamination, unplanned exposure, and costs associated with license termination and decommissioning activities, beginning with the application process for new licenses. Decommissioning means removing a facility or site safely from service and reducing residual radioactivity to a level that permits release of the property for unrestricted use and termination of the license. Information that the NRC considers important includes records of spills or other unusual occurrences involving the spread of contamination. These records may be limited to instances when contamination remains after any cleanup procedures.

Because of the low-activity inventory and short half-lives of byproduct materials used, diagnostic nuclear medicine facilities would not have to take any action beyond the usual procedures performed as part of their overall radiation protection programs. For example, most licensees use sealed sources authorized by 10 CFR Part 35 that usually pose minimal risk of radioactive contamination. Licensees are required to leak test these sealed sources, and these tests will demonstrate whether there has been any leakage of radioactive material. Leaking sources must be withdrawn from use immediately. These steps serve to minimize the spread of contamination and reduce radioactive waste associated with decontamination efforts.

Radioactive spills may occur from time to time, and personnel must know how to deal with such incidents. A spill procedure depends on many incident-specific variables, such as the number of individuals affected, likelihood of contamination spread, types and surfaces contaminated, and radiation hazard of the spilled material. In the practice of diagnostic nuclear medicine, these spills are usually minor radiation incidents. Although the NRC has no explicit requirements for spill procedures, the need for such procedures can be inferred from the general radiation protection program requirements under § 20.1101.

9.4.3 Suggested Procedures for Compliance

Contamination and the radioactive waste associated with decontamination efforts should be minimized to a large extent by the licensee's procedures, discussed elsewhere in Chapter 9 of this volume (e.g., sealed source leak testing, opening packages, control of airborne radiation levels, and radiation safety instruction to workers). In general, radiation workers should always monitor themselves for radioactive contamination before leaving restricted areas or the facility.

Regulatory Issues at a Glance
Minimization of Contamination/Spill Procedures

Design of facility

Minimization of contamination and generation of radioactive waste

Radioactive spills

9.4.3.1 Model Spill Procedure

(1) Notify all persons in the area that a spill has occurred.

(2) Prevent the spread of contamination by isolating the area and covering the spill, if appropriate, with absorbent paper. If clothing is contaminated, remove that article of clothing and place in a plastic bag. If an individual is contaminated, rinse contaminated area with lukewarm water and wash with a mild soap, using gloves.

(3) Notify the radiation safety officer or appropriate individual of any unusual circumstances immediately.

(4) Wearing gloves, a disposable lab coat, and booties, if necessary, clean up the spill with absorbent paper. Place absorbent paper and all other contaminated disposable material in appropriately labeled radioactive waste containers.

(5) Survey the area or contaminated individual with an appropriate radiation survey instrument, and check for removable contamination. If necessary, continue to decontaminate the area or individual until decontamination activities no longer result in reductions in removable activity. If necessary, leave absorbent paper labeled "Caution: Radioactive Material" over the area to prevent loosening of any fixed contamination. If necessary, shield the spill area to reduce ambient exposure levels.

(6) Check hands and clothing for self-contamination.

(7) Report the incident to the radiation safety officer or appropriate supervisory personnel. If personnel contamination is found, the skin dose will be evaluated.

In the case of a gas "spill," such as in a room in which ^{133}Xe is used, it is recommended that information be available that specifies the period of time for which the room should be evacuated, if necessary, after an accidental release of gas. In the event of an evacuation, without alarming the patient, instruct all individuals to leave the room as quickly as possible, making sure to close the door behind them to minimize leakage to surrounding unrestricted areas. The evacuation time can be based on the conservative occupational limit specified for a restricted area (i.e., a derived air concentration [DAC] of 1×10^{-4} μCi/mL for ^{133}Xe, as specified by the NRC in Table 1 of Appendix B to Part 20). The evacuation time (T, in minutes) is calculated as:

$$T = V/Q \ln (A/CV), \tag{9-15}$$

where V is the room air volume in milliliters (1 cubic foot [cft] ≅ 28,300 mL); Q is the total room air exhaust rate in mL/min; A is the released activity of ^{133}Xe in microcuries; and C is the restricted area DAC for ^{133}Xe (equal to 1×10^{-4} μCi/mL). Returning to the previous example, assuming room dimensions of 12 × 12 × 8 feet, an exhaust rate of 115.2 cft/min, and a gas "spill" involving the largest activity of ^{133}Xe used (20 mCi [740 MBq]), the room evacuation time would be:

$$V = 12 \times 12 \times 8 \text{ ft} \times 28{,}300 \text{ mL/cft} = 3.26 \times 10^7 \text{ mL}; \tag{9-16}$$

$$Q = 115.2 \text{ cft/min} \times 28{,}300 \text{ mL/cft} = 3.26 \times 10^6 \text{ mL/min}; \tag{9-17}$$

$$A = 20 \text{ mCi} = 2 \times 10^4 \ \mu\text{Ci}; \tag{9-18}$$

$$C = 1 \times 10^{-4} \ \mu\text{Ci/mL; and} \tag{9-19}$$

$$T = \frac{3.26 \times 10^7 \text{ mL}}{3.26 \times 10^6 \text{ mL/min}} \ln \left(\frac{2 \times 10^4 \ \mu\text{Ci}}{(1 \times 10^{-4} \ \mu\text{Ci/mL})(3.26 \times 10^7 \text{ mL})} \right) = 18 \text{ min.} \tag{9-20}$$

Licensees should perform this calculation for their specific facility layout and the maximum activity of ^{133}Xe likely to be used. (Note: Some licensees may choose not to evacuate the room, because the radiation dose is minimal from a "spill" of a standard activity administration of ^{133}Xe in a properly ventilated room. Licensees can use the information in section 9.2 to calculate the expected dose based on their facility design.)

Licensees should evaluate all spills to determine whether any corrective actions are necessary (e.g., modification of certain operating procedures, such as the need for more frequent area contamination surveys if spills are a frequent occurrence [see section 9.6]) or additional safety instruction.

9.5 Material Receipt and Accountability/Ordering, Receiving, and Opening Packages

9.5.1 Pertinent Regulations

10 CFR 20.1801 Security of stored material.
Licensee must secure from unauthorized removal or access licensed materials that are stored in controlled or unrestricted areas.

10 CFR 20.1802 Control of material not in storage.
Licensee must control and maintain constant surveillance of licensed material that is in a controlled or unrestricted area and that is not in storage.

10 CFR 20.1906 Procedures for receiving and opening packages.
Each licensee must monitor the external surfaces of a package labeled with a Radioactive White I, Yellow II, or Yellow III label for radioactive contamination. If there is evidence of degradation of integrity (e.g., the package is crushed, wet, or damaged), the

Material Receipt and Accountability/Ordering, Receiving, and Opening Packages

Pertinent regulations:

10 CFR 20.1801	Security of stored material.
10 CFR 20.1802	Control of material not in storage.
10 CFR 20.1906	Procedures for receiving and opening packages.

The complete text of these regulations can be accessed online through the NRC electronic reading room at www.nrc.gov.

TABLE 9.4
Radiation Level Limits by Package Label
(U.S. Department of Transportation Regulations)

Label type	Package surface limit*	1-meter limit (transport index)*
White I	0.5 mrem/h	0 mrem/h
Yellow II	50.0 mrem/h	1 mrem/h
Yellow III	200.0 mrem/h	10 mrem/h

*SI conversion: 1 mrem = 0.01 mSv.

package must be monitored for radioactive contamination and radiation levels. Monitoring must be performed as soon as practical after receipt of the package but no later than 3 hours after package receipt during normal working hours. If received at other times, the package must be monitored no later than 3 hours after the start of the next working day.

Licensee must immediately notify the final delivery carrier and the NRC Operations Center by telephone (301-816-5100) when any of the following levels exist:

(1) Radiation level >200 mrem/h (2 mSv/h) at any point on the surface or 10 mrem/h (100 Sv/h) at 1 meter (§ 71.47)

(2) Removable surface contamination >22 dpm/cm^2 for beta-and gamma-emitting radionuclides (§ 71.87 and 40 CFR 173.443).

Each licensee must establish, maintain, and retain written procedures for safely opening packages in which radioactive material is received and ensure that the procedures are followed.

9.5.2 Discussion of the Requirements

Each licensee must be able to account for all radioactive materials in their possession. Licensed materials must be tracked from "cradle to grave" to ensure accountability and identify circumstances in which licensed material could be lost, stolen, or misplaced. Each licensee must have written procedures for safely ordering, receiving, and opening packages in which radioactive material is received and ensure that the procedures are followed. Licensees exercise control over licensed material accountability by recording each dosage before medical use (see section 9.9), by performing physical inventories of sealed sources (see section 9.2), and when ordering and receiving licensed material. Licensees must ensure that the type and quantity of licensed material possessed is in accordance with the license and that packages are secured and radiation exposure from packages is minimized.

Radiation level limits for the various labeled packages as regulated by the U.S. Department of Transportation (49 CFR 172.403) are included in Table 9.4. Most packages received by a diagnostic nuclear medicine facility will have a White I or Yellow II label.

9.5.3 Suggested Procedures for Compliance

Licensed materials must be secured at all times, either by storage in a locked room (such as the hot lab) or by constant surveillance (such as in imaging rooms in which patient dosages may be located).

9.5.3.1 Model Procedure for Ordering and Receiving Packages Containing Radioactive Material

The purpose of these procedures is to ensure that ordered materials are authorized by the license and that upon receipt they will be accounted for and adequately secured.

(1) Each order of radioactive material will be authorized (e.g., by the authorized user or a supervised individual).

(2) Records will be kept that identify the facility and supplier and verify that ordered materials are authorized by the license for use (e.g., licensees authorized to use 35.200 materials may use any unsealed byproduct material prepared for medical use for imaging and localization studies that is appropriately obtained or prepared; no activity limit applies).

(3) For delivery during normal working hours, carriers will be informed to deliver radioactive packages directly to a specified area (generally the hot lab). For deliveries during off-duty hours, designated individuals will be instructed to accept and secure the "after hours" radioactive packages. These individuals also will be capable of determining whether packages are damaged. If the package is

Regulatory Issues at a Glance: Material Receipt and Accountability/Ordering, Receiving, and Opening Packages

Security of radioactive materials in storage
Security of radioactive materials not in storage
Receiving and opening packages

damaged, the carrier will not be allowed to leave and the specified responsible individual (radiation safety officer [RSO] or appropriate personnel) at the specified telephone or beeper number will be called. If a damaged package is received and contamination is found, the driver and the delivery vehicle will be surveyed for radioactive contamination as soon as the responsible individual is available.

9.5.3.2 Model Procedure for Safely Opening Packages Containing Radioactive Material

(1) Cover all areas in the hot lab at which packages will be received and opened, using disposable materials having plastic on one side and an absorbent material on the other. Wear gloves to prevent hand contamination.

(2) Check the user ordering request to ensure that the material received is the material ordered, and inspect packages visually for any signs of damage. This must be done within 3 hours of receipt during normal working hours and no later than 3 hours from the beginning of the next working day if the package was received after working hours. If damage is noted, stop and measure external radiation levels at 1 meter to determine whether the radiation limit for the package is exceeded (e.g., for White I-labeled package, the limit is 0 mrem/h). If so, notify the RSO or appropriate supervisory personnel. If not, measure the external radiation level at the surface and again determine if it is above the limit for the package (e.g., for White I-labeled package, limit is 0.5 mrem/h [5 μSv/h]). If so, notify the appropriate individual. The licensee will immediately notify the final delivery carrier and the NRC Operations Center (301-816-5100) if external radiation levels exceed 200 mrem/h (2 mSv/h) at any point on the surface or 10 mrem/h (0.1 mSv/h) at 1 meter. If not, continue.

(3) Monitor external surfaces of package for radioactive contamination. If a wipe sample indicates that removable radioactive contamination exceeds the applicable limit (i.e., 6,600 dpm for the wipe, based on a wiped surface area of 300 cm^2 with a removable contamination limit of 22 dpm/cm^2), notify the appropriate individual and determine if the package has contaminated any areas in the facility. The licensee will immediately notify the final delivery carrier and the NRC Operations Center (301-816-5100). If the wipe sample does not indicate contamination above the limits, continue.

(4) Remove the packing slip.

(5) Open the outer package, following any instructions that may be provided by the supplier.

(6) Open the inner package and verify that the contents agree with the packing slip.

(7) Check the integrity of the final source container. If there is any reason to suspect contamination, wipe external surface to determine if there is any removable radioactivity.

(8) Monitor the packing material and empty package with a radiation detection survey meter before discarding. If this material is contaminated, treat it as radioactive waste. If not, remove or obliterate the radiation labels before discarding in the normal trash or recycling.

(9) Make a record for each package and retain for at least 3 years.

9.6 Radiation Surveys and Calibration of Survey Instruments

9.6.1 Pertinent Regulations

10 CFR 20.1501 General.

Licensees must make or cause to be made, surveys that:

(1) May be necessary for the licensee to comply with Part 20 regulations; and

Radiation Surveys and Calibration of Survey Instruments

Pertinent regulations:

10 CFR 20.1501	General
10 CFR 35.61	Calibration of survey instruments

The complete text of these regulations can be accessed online through the NRC electronic reading room at www.nrc.gov.

(2) Are reasonable under the circumstance to evaluate:
  a. Magnitude and extent of radiation levels;
  b. Concentrations or quantities of radioactive material; and
  c. Potential radiological hazards.

The licensee must ensure that instruments and equipment used for quantitative radiation measurements (e.g., dose rate, radioactive contamination, and effluent monitoring) are calibrated periodically for the radiation measured.

10 CFR 35.61 Calibration of survey instruments. Licensees must calibrate survey instruments before first use, annually, and after repairs that affect the calibration.

9.6.2 Discussion of the Requirements

Licensees are required to perform surveys that are both necessary and reasonable. These surveys include the use of radiation detection or monitoring instruments to perform measurements of radiation or of concentrations of radioactive material (e.g., radiation survey instruments for external radiation levels and an appropriate wipe counter, such as a sodium iodide well scintillation counter, for evaluation of wipe survey levels of removable radioactive contamination). At least one portable survey instrument capable of detecting radiation levels from 0.1–100 mrem/h (1–1000 μSv/h) must be available at all times.

Regulatory Issues at a Glance: Radiation Surveys and Calibration of Survey Instruments

External dose rate surveys
Contamination (wipe) surveys
Proper instruments
Instrument calibration
Personnel knowledgeable in instrument operation

Radiation surveys are performed for a variety of purposes, such as personnel self-checking for radioactive contamination before leaving the facility, control of airborne radiation levels, testing after spills or other radiation incidents (see section 9.4), checking incoming packages containing radioactive materials (see section 9.5), sealed source leak testing (see section 9.10), and testing before waste disposal (see section 9.11). Additional routine surveys for determination of external radiation levels or removable radioactive contamination levels are not necessary or reasonable for those diagnostic nuclear medicine licensees who can demonstrate that: (1) workers are not likely to receive doses >10% of the applicable limits for internal or external exposure based on historical personnel dosimetry data; and (2) public doses are not likely to exceed applicable limits based on measurements or calculations demonstrating that the total effective dose equivalent (TEDE) to the individual member of the public likely to receive the highest dose does not exceed the annual dose limit of 100 mrem (1 mSv) (a reasonable estimate of public dose, presented in section 9.3, indicated that it is improbable for any member of the public to receive an annual radiation dose or dose rate in 1 hour that exceeds applicable dose limits). In this case, workers would not have to be issued individual monitoring devices and only the following surveys would be reasonable and necessary:

(1) Occasional surveys of radiation levels in work areas and unrestricted areas. Generally a survey with a Geiger-Mueller (GM) survey meter or other appropriately sensitive survey instrument for gross contamination and ambient levels of radiation would be considered sufficient. A thorough understanding of the radiation levels in work areas is desired. The frequency of these surveys is dependent on the variability and magnitude of the radiation levels as determined by the licensee's own prior experience based on reviews of its radiation protection program;
(2) Surveys after radioactive spills or other contamination incidents; and

(3) Surveys, as needed, after significant changes in regulations, terms of the license, procedures, or type of licensed material used.

Licensees must ensure that instruments used to measure radiation levels or determine radioactive contamination levels (e.g., dose rate or quantity of removable radioactive contamination) are capable of accurately detecting the radiation or radioactivity of interest. This is best accomplished by periodic calibration.

There are no requirements in the revised Part 35 or elsewhere describing the level of removable contamination that may serve as an action level for wipe surveys. Based on recommendations of the National Council on Radiation Protection and Measurements (NCRP), the International Atomic Energy Agency, the American National Standards Institute, and calculations performed by Vernig and Miron (*RSO Magazine.* 2000;4:1–7), removable contamination limits on the order of 18,000–400,000 dpm/100 cm^2 would be appropriate for ^{131}I, which is the highest risk radionuclide used in diagnostic nuclear medicine. These levels of radioactive contamination, if present and ingested, would result in negligible doses to workers and members of the public. To be conservative, a value of 22,000 dpm/100 cm^2 is suggested as a trigger level for wipe surveys.

9.6.3 Suggested Procedures for Compliance

Routine radiation surveys are performed for the following purposes: personnel checking themselves for radioactive contamination before leaving the facility (these surveys usually are not documented), checking incoming packages containing radioactive materials, sealed source leak testing, and testing before waste disposal. In addition, surveys must be performed after radioactive spills or other contamination incidents. These procedures are described elsewhere in this volume. Additional routine surveys for determination of external radiation levels or removable radioactive contamination levels are necessary or reasonable only if: (1) workers are likely to receive doses >10% of the applicable limits for internal or external exposure; and (2) public doses are likely to exceed applicable limits based on measurements or calculations demonstrating that the TEDE to the individual member of the public likely to receive the highest dose will exceed the annual dose limit of 100 mrem (1 mSv).

9.6.3.1 Model Procedure for Conducting Area Contamination Surveys

The purpose of this survey is to identify areas of radioactive contamination. Routine surveys of dose rates initially should be performed weekly with an appropriate survey meter in:

(1) Restricted areas, where workers may be exposed to radiation levels that might result in radiation doses >10% of the occupational dose limits; and

(2) Unrestricted areas, where members of the public may be exposed to radiation levels that might result in radiation doses that exceed the public dose limits.

Some licensees may feel more comfortable performing daily area surveys. In such circumstances, these surveys need only be documented on a weekly basis. For established licensees with prior experience that demonstrates that no worker or member of the public is likely to receive a dose in excess of the applicable limits, only occasional radiation surveys should be performed monthly or at even longer intervals, if justified by historical survey data. This change to the radiation protection program must first be reviewed and approved by the radiation safety officer (RSO) and licensee management. All affected individuals will be instructed on the revised program. (There is no need for NRC approval in the form of a license amendment [§ 35.26].) As an alternative to radiation surveys in unrestricted areas, licensees may choose to demonstrate compliance with the dose limits for members of the public, pursuant to 10 CFR 20.1301 and 1302 (see section 9.3), by placement of long-term dosimeters, such as film badges, in areas of concern.

Radiation surveys must be performed with a sufficiently sensitive survey meter. Personnel must be familiar with proper operation of the instrument and must know what procedures to follow in the event that the equipment is not functioning properly. The RSO or appropriate supervisory personnel must be notified if established radiation levels are exceeded in restricted or unrestricted areas. (Trigger levels will be set at 5.0 mrem/h [50 μSv] and 0.2 mrem/h [2 μSv] in restricted and unrestricted areas, respectively.). After significant changes in regulations, terms of the license, procedures, or the type of licensed material used, after new personnel are hired, and/or if radioactive contamination is a frequent occurrence (see section 9.4), the current survey frequency can be modified. More frequent surveys should be performed until such time that experience demonstrates that a more infrequent schedule may be resumed.

9.6.3.2 Model Procedure for Conducting Removable Contamination (Wipe) Surveys

Routine contamination surveys should initially be performed weekly in:

(1) Restricted areas, where workers may be exposed to radioactive contamination levels that might result in radiation doses >10% of the occupational dose limits; and

(2) Unrestricted areas, where members of the public may be exposed to radioactive contamination levels that might result in radiation doses that exceed public dose limits.

For established licensees with prior experience that demonstrates that no worker or member of the public is likely to receive a dose in excess of the applicable limits, only occasional contamination surveys should be performed (monthly, quarterly, or at even longer intervals if justified by historical wipe survey data). Some established licensees may choose not to perform contamination surveys at all unless spills occur or area surveys reveal the presence of radioactive contamination. This change to the radiation protection program would need to be reviewed and approved by the RSO and licensee management. All affected individuals must also be instructed about the revised program (There is no need for NRC approval in the form of a license amendment [§ 35.26].)

These surveys must be analyzed with an appropriate detector system, such as a sodium iodide well scintillation counter (a shielded GM probe or uncollimated gamma camera also may be used for this purpose). The RSO or appropriate supervisory personnel will be notified if established radioactive contamination levels are exceeded in restricted or unrestricted areas (the contamination trigger level will be set at 22,000 dpm/ $100cm^2$).

Additional wipe surveys should be performed after spills or other radiation incidents. After significant changes in regulations, terms of the license, procedures, or type of licensed material used, and/or after new personnel are hired, the current wipe survey frequency may require modification. More frequent surveys may have to be performed until such time as experience demonstrates otherwise. All contamination surveys should be recorded.

Internal radiation contamination in individuals working in areas where unsealed radioactive materials are used should be minimized by simple radiation safety practices. Procedures to handle and minimize intake of radioactive materials should be followed by all workers when they are in any area where radioactive materials are used or stored. These procedures include:

(1) Wearing laboratory coats or other protective clothing;

(2) Using disposable gloves;

(3) Not eating, drinking, smoking, inserting or removing contact lenses, or applying cosmetics;

(4) Not storing food, drink, or personal items;

(5) Never pipetting by mouth; and

(6) Monitoring hands and body for contamination when leaving.

9.6.3.3 Calibration of Survey Instruments

Diagnostic nuclear medicine licensees usually send their dose-rate instruments back to the manufacturer, supplier, or commercial service for calibration. During this calibration period, licensees who do not possess a spare must obtain an appropriately calibrated loaner instrument for use until their instrument is returned. Instruments should be calibrated before first use, annually, and after repairs that affect calibration. The licensee must keep a copy of the calibration results for each survey instrument.

9.6.3.4 Calibration of Sodium Iodide Well Scintillation Counter

The well counter must be calibrated by determining the detector efficiency. The detector efficiency is the efficiency of the well counter as determined by assaying a standard check source (std) of either the same radionuclide as the source being tested or one with similar energy characteristics. The activity of each check source must be certified by the supplier. The detector efficiency or efficiencies necessary to determine radioactive contamination from any radionuclide used in diagnostic nuclear medicine (or for any sealed source required to be tested for leakage) must be determined and recorded at least annually. Detector efficiency is calculated as follows:

$$\textbf{Detector efficiency} = \frac{\textbf{Measured std activity (cpm) – background (cpm)}}{\textbf{Std activity } (\mu\textbf{Ci})(2.22 \text{ ¥ } 10^6 \textbf{ dpm}/\mu\textbf{Ci})} \quad (9\text{-}21)$$

The well counter must be calibrated before first use, annually, and after repairs. The licensee must keep a copy of the calibration results.

9.7 Caution Signs and Posting Requirements

9.7.1 Pertinent Regulations

10 CFR 19.11 Posting of notices to workers.

Licensees must either post current copies or a notice (describing content and location) of all of the following:

(1) 10 CFR Parts 19 and 20;

(2) License and related documents;

(3) Operating procedures applicable to licensed activities;

(4) Notices of violation, penalties, or orders and any licensee response; and

(5) NRC Form 3, *Notice to Employees.*

All postings must be in a sufficient number of places to permit their review. These postings must be conspicuous and replaced if defaced or altered. Any documents posted pursuant to item 4 in the previous list must be posted within 2 working days after receipt or transmittal and remain posted for a minimum of 5 working days or until corrective actions are completed (whichever is later).

Caution Signs and Posting Requirements

Pertinent regulations:

10 CFR 19.11	Posting of notices to workers
10 CFR 20.1901	Caution signs
10 CFR 20.1902	Posting requirements
10 CFR 20.1903	Exceptions to posting requirements

The complete text of these regulations can be accessed online through the NRC electronic reading room at www.nrc.gov.

10 CFR 20.1901 Caution signs.

The standard radiation symbol must be used. Additional pertinent information may be added on or near these signs to make individuals aware of potential radiation exposures and to minimize these exposures.

10 CFR 20.1902 Posting requirements.

All areas in which radioactive materials are stored or used in excess of 10 times the quantity specified in 10 CFR Part 20, Appendix C, must be posted with a sign bearing the radiation symbol and the words CAUTION (or DANGER), RADIOACTIVE MATERIAL(S). Areas where individuals could receive a dose equivalent >5 mrem (50 μSv) in 1 hour at 30 cm from the source must also be posted with a sign bearing the radiation symbol and the words CAUTION RADIATION AREA.

The licensee must post each airborne radioactivity area with a conspicuous sign bearing the radiation symbol and the words CAUTION (or DANGER), AIRBORNE RADIOACTIVITY AREA.

10 CFR 20.1903 Exceptions to posting requirements.

A licensee is not required to post caution signs in areas or rooms that contain radioactive materials if any of the following are met:

(1) Materials are contained in an area under licensee control for <8 hours and are constantly attended by an individual who takes precautions to prevent overexposures;

(2) Radiation exposure from a patient who can be released pursuant to § 35.75; or

(3) Radiation exposure from a sealed source measuring 5 mrem/h (50 μSv/h) or less at 30 cm.

9.7.2 Discussion of the Requirements

Certain areas (i.e., restricted areas) within a diagnostic nuclear medicine facility must be posted with warning signs. These postings should serve as warnings to individuals of specific radiological hazards; overposting will detract from this intent. The NRC recognizes that, in certain circumstances, posting may not be necessary. For example, licensees are not required to post caution signs in areas where byproduct material is contained for short periods of time (<8 h/day) if these areas are constantly attended by someone adequately trained to take precautions necessary to prevent exposure of individuals to radioactive materials. Typically, the only locations in a diagnostic nuclear medicine facility that require posting are the hot lab, the decay storage area, and the patient imaging room(s). If imaging rooms are used for <8 h/day and are constantly attended, no posting is required.

Many diagnostic nuclear medicine licensees typically use ^{133}Xe in gaseous form to perform lung scintigraphy for pulmonary embolism. According to Part 20, an airborne radioactivity area means an area in which airborne radioactive materials exist in concentrations in excess of the derived air concentrations (DACs) specified in Appendix B of Part 20 or to such a degree that an individual present in the area without respiratory protection could exceed, during the hours an individual is present in a week, an intake of 0.6% of the annual limit on intake or 12 DAC-hours (DAC-h). This is equivalent to a committed effective dose equivalent (CEDE) of 30 mrem (0.3 mSv). These two conditions are only equivalent if an individual remains in the area for 12 h/wk. Because it is likely that a worker (e.g., nuclear medicine technologist) may be in the area for 40 h/wk (i.e., 40 DAC-h), the latter condition applies. Because ^{133}Xe poses an external rather than an internal hazard, the DAC is calculated directly from the external dose, assuming immersion in a semi-infinite cloud of the gas. As stated in section 9.2, the external dose is best assessed by radiation dose measurements using personnel dosimeters. Nevertheless, it is possible to calculate whether the example ^{133}Xe room described in section 9.2 would be considered an airborne radioactivity area. Assuming a room air exhaust rate of 115.2 cubic feet per minute (cfm), an average air concentration of radioactivity (C) of 2.6×10^{-6} μCi/mL, the fact that a DAC-hour is the product of C/DAC (i.e., the estimated average air concentration of radioactive material divided by the DAC of 1×10^{-4} μCi/mL for ^{133}Xe), and the time of exposure in hours, it is only necessary to demonstrate that:

$$\mathbf{C \times 40\ h/DAC < 12\ DAC\text{-}h,} \quad (9\text{-}22)$$

in order not to be required to post the room as an airborne radioactivity area. Because:

$$\mathbf{C \times 40/DAC = \frac{2.6 \times 10^{-6}\ \mu Ci/mL \times 40\ hours}{1 \times 10^{-4}\ \mu Ci/mL} = 1.04\ DAC\text{-}h,} \quad (9\text{-}23)$$

And:

$$\mathbf{1.04\ DAC\text{-}h < 12\ DAC\text{-}h,} \quad (9\text{-}24)$$

our example room need not be posted.

For hospitals, 10 CFR Part 35.75 allows licensees to release patients containing radiopharmaceuticals when the dose to any other individual is not likely to exceed 0.5 rem (5 mSv). For this reason, rooms occupied by these patients would not need to be posted if the person is hospitalized for some reason unrelated to the radioactivity. However, some licensees may choose to take this precaution to minimize dose as part of their as low as reasonably achievable procedures.

Regulatory Issues at a Glance: Caution Signs and Posting Requirements

Posting of required documents or notices
Caution signs
Posting requirements

9.7.3 Suggested Procedures for Compliance

The licensee must post current copies or a notice (describing content and location) of all of the following:

(1) 10 CFR Parts 19 and 20;
(2) License and related documents;
(3) Operating procedures applicable to licensed activities;
(4) Notices of violation, penalties, or orders and any licensee response; and
(5) NRC Form 3, *Notice to Employees.*

The licensee must post in all areas in which radioactive materials are stored or used in excess of 10 times the quantity specified in 10 CFR 20, Appendix C (see section 9.13 of this chapter), a sign bearing the radiation symbol and the words CAUTION (or DANGER), RADIOACTIVE MATERIAL(S) and an additional sign bearing the radiation symbol and the words CAUTION

RADIATION AREA. Such signs must be posted in all areas where it is possible for an individual to receive a dose >5 mrem (0.05 mSv) in any 1 hour.

Licensees need not post the sign bearing the radiation symbol and the words CAUTION (or DANGER), AIRBORNE RADIOACTIVITY AREA in areas in which ^{133}Xe is employed, unless considerations of room size, workload, activity release, and/or room ventilation rates indicate otherwise.

9.8 Labeling Containers, Vials, and Syringes

9.8.1 Pertinent Regulations

10 CFR 20.1904 Labeling containers.

Licensees must ensure that each container of licensed material is labeled with the radiation symbol and the words CAUTION (or DANGER), RADIOACTIVE MATERIAL. The label must also provide sufficient information (such as radionuclide and quantity of radioactivity at a specified date and time) to permit individuals handling or using the containers or working in the vicinity of the containers to take precautions to avoid or minimize exposures.

Licensees must remove or deface the radioactive material label or otherwise clearly indicate that the container no longer contains radioactive materials before removal or disposal of empty uncontaminated containers to unrestricted areas.

10 CFR 32.72 Manufacture, preparation, or transfer for commercial distribution of radioactive drugs containing byproduct material for medical use under part 35.

Licensees who manufacture, prepare, or transfer for commercial distribution radioactive drugs containing byproduct material must satisfy the following two labeling requirements:

(1) A label must be affixed to each transport radiation shield and include the radiation symbol and the words CAUTION (or DANGER), RADIOACTIVE MATERIAL, the name of the radioactive drug, and the quantity of radioactivity at a specified date and time; and

(2) A label must be affixed to each syringe, vial, or other container and include the radiation symbol and the words CAUTION (or DANGER), RADIOACTIVE MATERIAL, and an identifier that ensures that the container can be correlated with the information on the transport radiation shield label.

10 CFR 35.69 Labeling of vials and syringes.

Each syringe or vial that contains unsealed byproduct material must be labeled to identify the radioactive drug. Each syringe shield and vial shield also must be labeled, unless the label on the syringe or vial is visible when shielded.

Labeling Containers, Vials, and Syringes

Pertinent regulations:

10 CFR 20.1904	Labeling containers
10 CFR 32.72	Manufacture, preparation, or transfer for commercial distribution of radioactive drugs containing byproduct material for medical use under part 35
10 CFR 35.69	Labeling of vials and syringes

The complete text of these regulations can be accessed online through the NRC electronic reading room at www.nrc.gov.

9.8.2 Discussion of the Requirements

Adequate information must be available to workers to enable them to handle radioactive materials safely, minimize exposure, and ensure that the proper material is administered to all patients. It is important to remove or deface radioactive material labels on empty uncontaminated containers, because, if found in the public domain, these labels may cause undue alarm on the part of the public and have an impact on the radiation safety resources of licensees and regulatory agencies.

9.8.3 Suggested Procedures for Compliance

Licensees must ensure that each container of licensed

Regulatory Issues at a Glance: Labeling Containers, Vials, and Syringes

- Labeling containers
- Labeling vials and syringes
- Syringe and vial shields

material is labeled with the radiation symbol and the words CAUTION (or DANGER), RADIOACTIVE MATERIAL. The label also must provide the radionuclide and quantity of radioactivity at a specified date and time.

Licensees must remove or deface the radioactive material label or otherwise clearly indicate that the container no longer contains radioactive materials before removal or disposal of empty uncontaminated containers to unrestricted areas.

Each syringe or vial that contains unsealed byproduct material must be labeled to identify the radioactive agent. Each syringe shield and vial shield, if necessary, also must be labeled, unless the label on the syringe or vial is visible when shielded.

9.9 Determining Patient Dosages

9.9.1 Pertinent Regulations

10 CFR 35.60 Possession, use, and calibration of instruments used to measure the activity of unsealed byproduct material.

If direct measurements are required under § 35.63, licensees must possess and use instrumentation to measure the activity of unsealed byproduct material before it is administered to each patient or human research subject.

Licensees must calibrate the instrumentation and record the results in accordance with nationally recognized standards or the manufacturer's instructions.

10 CFR 35.63 Determination of dosages of unsealed byproduct material for medical use.

Licensees must determine and record the activity of each dosage before medical use. For a unit dosage, this determination can by made by

(1) Direct measurement; or
(2) Decay correction based on the activity (or activity concentration) determined by an appropriately licensed manufacturer or preparer or a recognized licensee for use in research in accordance with a Radioactive Drug Research Committee (RDRC)-approved protocol or an Investigational New Drug (IND) protocol accepted by the U.S. Food and Drug Administration (FDA).

Determining Patient Dosages

Pertinent regulations:

10 CFR 35.60	Possession, use, and calibration of instruments used to measure the activity of unsealed byproduct material.
10 CFR 35.63	Determination of dosages of unsealed byproduct material for medical use.
10 CFR 35.204	Permissible ^{99}Mo concentration.

The complete text of these regulations can be accessed online through the NRC electronic reading room at www.nrc.gov.

Note: NRC defines unit dosage as "a dosage prepared for medical use for administration as a single dosage to a patient or human research subject without any further manipulation of the dosage after it is initially prepared."

For other than unit dosages, this determination can be made by:

(1) Direct measurement;
(2) Combination of measurement and mathematical calculations; or
(3) Combination of volumetric measurements and mathematical calculations, based on measurement determined by an appropriately licensed manufacturer or preparer.

Unless otherwise directed by the authorized user (AU), a licensee may not use a dosage if the dosage does not fall within the prescribed dosage range or if the dosage differs from the prescribed dosage by >20%.

10 CFR 35.204 Permissible ^{99}Mo concentration.

Licensees may not administer to humans a radiopharmaceutical that contains >0.15 μCi ^{99}Mo/mCi ^{99m}Tc (>0.15 kBq ^{99}Mo/MBq ^{99m}Tc).

Licensees using ^{99}Mo/^{99m}Tc generators must measure and record the ^{99}Mo concentration of the first eluate after receipt of a generator.

9.9.2 Discussion of the Requirements

Licensees must determine and record the activity of each dosage before medical use, even if it comes from a licensed radiopharmacy. Note that this requirement differs from that for all other drugs prepared and dispensed by licensed pharmacists and manufacturers. For all other drugs, it is not necessary for a physician to determine and/or record the weight of the active drug ingredients.

The hot lab is used to receive, store, and/or prepare radiopharmaceuticals that are administered to patients for nuclear medicine studies. An important component of the hot lab is the dose calibrator (or dosage calibrator, in NRC parlance), which measures radioactivity in vials, syringes, capsules, etc. It consists of a cylindrical, gas-filled detector (ionization chamber) and a readout device. The detector is often placed behind a lead or leaded-glass shield to minimize radiation exposure to the individual (e.g., technologist or radiopharmacist) while working with radioactivity. Patient dosages and shielded vials are also generally placed and/or stored behind this shield. It should be noted that unless diagnostic nuclear medicine licensees use a ^{99}Mo/^{99m}Tc generator or prepare their own patient dosages (rather than receiving them from a commercial radiopharmacy), they are not required to directly measure the activity of each dosage before medical use and, therefore, are not required to have a dose calibrator or other instrument capable of measuring radioactivity. Unit dosages of ^{99m}Tc from commercial radiopharmacies should be delivered with a label indicating that the molybdenum/technetium activity ratio is acceptable until a specified expiration time to preclude the need for a dose calibrator for this purpose. It must be emphasized that it is now a licensee's choice whether to use a dose calibrator. Because of historical reasons or other concerns, some licensees may be uncomfortable not using a dose calibrator.

AUs are responsible for prescribing the dosage or dosage range (a prescribed dosage is defined by the NRC as the specified activity or range of activity in accordance with the directions of the AU for diagnostic procedures). AUs may prescribe a dosage range >20%. This range can be case specific or can be a "blanket" range that would cover all administrations. For example, the AU could establish a policy whereby all administered dosage, could deviate from the prescribed dosage by plus or minus a specified percentage. The NRC does not allow a deviation outside the ±20%, because the AU has the flexibility of establishing the acceptable range under this provision. In cases in which the AU has not established a prescribed dosage range but rather a prescribed dosage, the 20% deviation will apply.

9.9.3 Suggested Procedures for Compliance

Diagnostic nuclear medicine licensees who receive all their dosages from an appropriately licensed manufacturer or preparer or a recognized licensee for use in research in accordance with RDRC-approved protocol or an IND protocol accepted by the FDA are not required to have a dose calibrator. In this case, the activity of each dosage must be determined (and recorded) by decay correction activity or a combination of volumetric measurements and mathematical calculations (based on the supplied activity measurement) before administration. Licensees must note the expiration time for ^{99m}Tc-labeled radiopharmaceuticals, which must not be administered past their expiration time. Licensees planning to conduct research involving human subjects should refer to § 35.6, *Provisions for the protection of human research subjects.* (Of course, if licensees so desire, they certainly can use the dose calibrator to directly measure the activity; in this case, the licensee is required to follow the procedures given in the following paragraph.)

Diagnostic nuclear medicine licensees that use a ^{99}Mo/^{99m}Tc generator or prepare their own dosages are required to determine and record the activity of each dosage before medical use by direct measurement. In this case, a dose calibrator must be employed for the activity determination and required recordkeeping as follows:

(1) ^{99}Mo activity present in any ^{99m}Tc preparation must be determined. It must be ≤ 0.15 μCi ^{99}Mo/mCi ^{99m}Tc (0.15 kBq ^{99}Mo/MBq ^{99m}Tc). If this activity ratio is exceeded, the dosage cannot be administered.

(2) ^{99}Mo concentration of the first eluate after receipt of a ^{99}Mo/^{99m}Tc generator must be measured and recorded.

Regulatory Issues at a Glance: Determining Patient Dosages

Determination of dosages for medical use
Requirement for dose calibrator
Required procedures with or without dose calibrator

(3) The dose calibrator must be calibrated, and the results recorded in accordance with nationally recognized standards or the manufacturer's instructions.

Personnel must be familiar with proper operation of the dose calibrator and know what actions to take in the event that the dose calibrator is nonfunctional. For example, in this case, the licensee may decide to switch to unit dosages because there is no regulation that requires a backup dose calibrator.

The authorized user physician should establish a policy for the prescribed dosage or dosage range. This prescribed dosage may be allowed to vary by plus or minus a specified percentage or a range could be established that could be case specific or cover all administrations. For example, the AU could establish a policy whereby all administered dosages could deviate from the prescribed dosage by ±50% or be in a range of 1–30 mCi (37–1,110 MBq). More specifically, a department's procedure manual for a bone scan could specify a typical administered dose of 20 mCi (740 mBq) with an acceptable range of 1–30 mCi (37–1,110 MBq).

9.10 Sealed Source Inventory and Leak Testing

9.10.1 Pertinent Regulations

10 CFR 35.65 Authorization for calibration, transmission, and reference sources.

Licensees may receive, possess, and use any of the following for check, calibration, transmission, and reference use:

(1) Sealed sources, not exceeding 30 mCi (1.11 GBq) each, manufactured and distributed by an appropriately licensed person;

(2) Any byproduct material with a half-life not longer than 120 days in individual amounts not exceeding 15 mCi (0.56 GBq);

(3) Any byproduct material with a half-life >120 days in individual amounts not exceeding the smaller of 200 μCi (7.4 MBq) or 1,000 times the quantities in Appendix B of Part 30; or

(4) ^{99m}Tc in amounts as needed.

10 CFR 35.67 Requirements for possession of sealed sources.

Licensees in possession of any sealed source must follow the radiation safety and handling instructions supplied by the manufacturer. Licensees in possession of a sealed source must:

(1) Test the source for leakage before its first use, unless tested within 6 months before transfer to licensee; and

(2) Test (and record) the source for leakage at intervals not to exceed 6 months; leak test must be capable of detecting 0.005 μCi (185 Bq).

If the leak test reveals the presence of >0.005 μCi (185 Bq) of removable contamination, the licensee must immediately withdraw the source from use and store, dispose, or cause it to be repaired. A report must be filed within 5 days.

Licensees are not required to perform a leak test on the following sources:

(1) Sources containing material with a half-life <30 days;

(2) Sources containing only gaseous material;

(3) Sources containing 100 μCi (3.7 MBq) or less of beta- or gamma-emitting material; or

(4) Sources stored and not being used.

Licensees must conduct a semiannual physical inventory of all sealed sources in their possession.

Sealed Source Inventory and Leak Testing

Pertinent regulations:

10 CFR 35.65	Authorization for calibration, transmission, and reference sources
10 CFR 35.67	Requirements for possession of sealed sources

The complete text of these regulations can be accessed online through the NRC electronic reading room at www.nrc.gov.

9.10.2 Discussion of the Requirements

Leak testing is an effective means of evaluating the integrity of a sealed source and minimizing the potential spread of radioactive contamination. Although NRC regulations pertain only to byproduct material, a well-managed safety program would leak test all sealed sources. Diagnostic nuclear medicine licensees, for the most part, use sealed sources that pose minimal risk of radioactive contamination.

Regulatory Issues at a Glance: Sealed Source Inventory and Leak Testing

Authorization for calibration, transmission, and reference sources
Requirements for possession of sealed sources
Inventory
Leak testing

Licensees are required to inventory and leak test these sealed sources. Leaking sources must be immediately withdrawn from use. These steps serve to minimize the spread of contamination and reduce radioactive waste associated with decontamination efforts.

9.10.3 Suggested Procedures for Compliance

The licensee must inventory, by listing on a semiannual basis, all sealed sources in its possession. Their locations (typically the hot lab) must also be recorded. The inventory record must contain the model number of each source and serial number (if one has been assigned), the identity of each source by radionuclide and its nominal activity, the location of each source, and the name of the individual who performed the inventory. Inventory records should be maintained for 3 years.

The licensee must wipe for removable radioactive contamination all sealed sources in its possession that are required to be tested for leakage at intervals not to exceed 6 months. (These will usually be the ^{57}Co flood source and the ^{57}Co and ^{137}Cs check sources for the dose calibrator; see section 9.10 for the necessity of dose calibrator). The following procedure should be used:

(1) A separate wipe sample (e.g., cotton swab, injection prep pad, or filter or tissue paper) should be obtained from each sealed source and appropriately identified. The individual performing the wipes must wear gloves and proper protective clothing.

(2) Each wipe sample should be counted for 1 minute in a sodium iodide well scintillation counter to obtain the wipe counts per minute (cpm) and recorded. A separate background count rate should also be obtained and recorded.

(3) The activity (in microcuries) of each wipe sample should then be determined according to:

$$\text{Activity } (\mu\text{Ci}) = \frac{\text{Measured wipe (cpm)} - \text{background (cpm)}}{\text{Detector efficiency} \times 2.22 \times 10^{6}\ \text{dpm}/\mu\text{Ci}}, \quad (9\text{-}25)$$

where detector efficiency is the efficiency of the well counter (see section 9.6 for determination of detector efficiency).

(4) Record activity in microcuries of each wipe sample. It must be <0.005 μCi. If not, the leaking source must be removed from use and stored, disposed, or caused to be repaired. A report must be filed within 5 days in accordance with § 35.3067.

(5) The leak test results must be recorded and must include the model number and serial number (if one has been assigned) of each source tested, the identity of each source by radionuclide and its estimated activity, the results of the test, the date of the test, the name of the individual who performed the test, and any action taken.

9.11 Waste Disposal and Decay-in-Storage

9.11.1 Pertinent Regulations

10 CFR 20.2001 General requirements.
Licensees are given four options for disposal of licensed material. For diagnostic nuclear medicine licensees, the method generally used is the NRC-approved option of decay-in-storage.

10 CFR 35.92 Decay-in-storage.
A licensee may hold byproduct material with physical half-lives of <120 days for decay-in-storage before disposal without regard to radioactivity if it:

Waste Disposal and Decay-In-Storage

Pertinent regulations:

10 CFR 20.2001	General requirements
10 CFR 35.92	Decay-in-storage

The complete text of these regulations can be accessed online through the NRC electronic reading room at www.nrc.gov.

(1) Monitors material at surface with an appropriate radiation detection survey meter set on its most sensitive scale with no interposed shielding before disposal and determines that its radioactivity cannot be distinguished from the background radiation levels; and

(2) Removes or obliterates all radiation labels, except for radiation labels on materials that are within containers and that will be managed as biomedical waste after they have been released from the licensee.

Licensees must retain a record of each permitted disposal in accordance with § 35.2092.

9.11.2 Discussion of the Requirements

Decay-in-storage, an effective alternative to low-level waste burial, means that the material is stored at the licensee's facility for a period sufficiently long to ensure that the activity decays to levels that permit disposal of the material as ordinary, nonradioactive waste. Disposal is permitted only after surveys demonstrate no detectable radioactivity (i.e., material must be indistinguishable from background radiation levels). Before disposal, the material must be stored in a manner that ensures radiological safety for the workers and the general public.

9.11.3 Suggested Procedures for Compliance

Storage could be designed to allow for segregation of wastes with different half-lives (e.g., different containers for short- and long-half-lived materials). Containers should be shielded and stored in a secure location (e.g., hot lab). The licensee must:

(1) Use separate containers, if possible, for different types of waste (e.g., needles and syringes in one container, swabs and gauze in another, unused dosages in a third).

(2) Seal the container when it is full and attach an identification tag that includes the date sealed and the longest-lived radionuclide in the container. The container may then be transferred to the decay-in-storage area if applicable.

(3) Before disposal as regular waste, monitor and record the results of monitoring for each container as follows:

Regulatory Issues at a Glance: Waste Disposal and Decay-In-Storage

Radioactive waste containers
Decay-in-storage
Molybdenum/technetium generators
Security and accountability

a. Use an appropriate survey instrument.

b. Remove any shielding from around the container.

c. Monitor, in a low-level radiation area if possible, all surfaces of each container.

d. Remove or deface any radioactive material labels. (Note: Sharps boxes are not to be opened to check for and/or to remove any labels that may be affixed to syringes, vials, etc., already contained in the box. The box should remain closed, and all radiation labels on the box must be removed or defaced before disposal.)

e. Discard as regular in-house waste, recycling, or infectious waste, as appropriate, only those containers that cannot be distinguished from background. Record the disposal date, the survey instrument used, the background radiation level, the radiation level measured at the surface of each waste container, and the name of the individual who performed the survey.

f. Return containers that can be distinguished from background radiation levels to the storage area for further decay.

The previous procedure is for decay-in-storage. If licensees use $^{99}Mo/^{99m}Tc$ generators, these may be returned to the manufacturer. In this case, the licensee must follow all applicable regulations when returning generators.

9.12 Records

9.12.1 Pertinent Regulations

10 CFR 20.2102 Records of radiation protection programs. Records of the provisions of the radiation protection program must be retained until license termination.

Records of audits and other reviews of program content and implementation must be retained for 3 years.

10 CFR 20.2103 Records of surveys.

Records showing the results of surveys and calibrations must be retained for 3 years. The following records must be retained until the license is terminated: records of surveys to determine the dose from external sources, records of measurements and calculations used to determine individual intakes of radioactive material and used in the assessment of internal dose, and records of measurements and calculations used to evaluate the release of radioactive effluents to the environment.

10 CFR 20.2106 Records of individual monitoring results.

Records of doses received by all individuals for whom monitoring was required must be maintained until license termination. The records must be made at least annually on NRC Form 5 or in clear and legible records (e.g., dosimetry processor's report) containing all the information required by NRC Form 5.

10 CFR 20.2107 Records of dose to individual members of the public.

Records sufficient to demonstrate compliance with the dose limit for individual members of the public must be retained until the license is terminated.

10 CFR 30.51 Records.

Records must be kept, showing the receipt, transfer, and disposal of byproduct material. Records of receipts must be kept for as long as the material is possessed and for 3 years following transfer or disposal. Records of disposal must be retained until license termination.

10 CFR 35.2024 Records of authority and responsibilities for radiation protection programs.

Records of actions taken by the licensee's management must be retained for 5 years and must include a summary of the actions taken, signed by licensee management. Copy of authority, duties, and responsibilities of the radiation safety officer (RSO) and a signed copy of each RSO's agreement to be responsible for implementing the radiation safety program must be retained for the duration of the license. The records must include signatures of the RSO and licensee management.

Records

Pertinent regulations:

10 CFR 20.2102	Records of radiation protection programs
10 CFR 20.2103	Records of surveys
10 CFR 20.2106	Records of individual monitoring results
10 CFR 20.2107	Records of dose to individual members of the public
10 CFR 30.51	Records
10 CFR 35.2024	Records of authority and responsibilities for radiation protection programs
10 CFR 35.2026	Records of radiation protection program changes
10 CFR 35.2060	Records of calibrations of instruments used to measure the activity of unsealed byproduct material
10 CFR 35.2061	Records of radiation survey instrument calibrations
10 CFR 35.2063	Records of dosages of unsealed byproduct material for medical use
10 CFR 35.2067	Records of leak tests and inventory of sealed sources
10 CFR 35.2080	Records of mobile medical services (if applicable)
10 CFR 35.2092	Records of decay-in-storage
10 CFR 35.2204	Records of ^{99}Mo concentrations

The complete text of these regulations can be accessed online through the NRC electronic reading room at www.nrc.gov.

10 CFR 35.2026 Records of radiation protection program changes.

Records of each radiation protection program change must be retained for 5 years and must include a copy of the old and new procedures, the effective date of the change, and the signature of the licensee management that reviewed and approved the change.

10 CFR 35.2060 Records of calibrations of instruments used to measure the activity of unsealed byproduct material.

Records of instrument calibrations must be maintained for 3 years and must include the model and serial number of the instrument, the date of the calibration, the results of the calibration, and the name of the individual who performed the calibration.

10 CFR 35.2061 Records of radiation survey instrument calibrations.

Records of radiation survey instrument calibrations must be maintained for 3 years and must include the model and serial number of the instrument, the date of the calibration, the results of the calibration, and the name of the individual who performed the calibration.

10 CFR 35.2063 Records of dosages of unsealed byproduct material for medical use.

Records of dosage determinations must be maintained for 3 years and must contain the radiopharmaceutical, the patient's or human research subject's name or identification number (if one has been assigned), the prescribed dosage, the determined dosage (or a notation that the total activity is <30 μCi [1.1 MBq]), the date and time of the dosage determination, and the name of the individual who determined the dosage.

10 CFR 35.2067 Records of leak tests and inventory of sealed sources.

Records of leak tests must be retained for 3 years and must include the model number and serial number (if one has been assigned) of each source tested, the identity of each source by radionuclide and its estimated activity, the results of the test, the date of the test, and the name of the individual who performed the test.

Records of the semiannual physical inventory of sealed sources must be retained for 3 years and must contain the model number of each source and serial number (if one has been assigned), the identity of each source by radionuclide and its nominal activity, the location of each source, and the name of the individual who performed the inventory.

10 CFR 35.2080 Records of mobile medical services (if applicable).

A copy of each letter signed by management of each client for which services are rendered that permits the use of byproduct material at a client's address must be retained for 3 years after the last provision of service and must clearly delineate the authority and responsibility of the licensee and the client.

Records of each survey must be retained for 3 years and must include the date of the survey, the results of the survey, the instrument used to make the survey, and the name of the individual who performed the survey.

Regulatory Issues at a Glance: Records

Appropriate records

- Radiation protection program
- Surveys
- Individual monitoring results
- Dose to individual members of the public
- Receipt, transfer, and disposal of byproduct material.
- Authority and responsibilities for radiation protection program
- Radiation protection program changes
- Calibrations of instruments used to measure activity of license material
- Radiation survey instrument calibrations
- Dosages of licensed material for medical use
- Leak test and inventory of sealed sources
- Mobile medical services (if applicable)
- Decay-in-storage
- ^{99}Mo concentration

10 CFR 35.2092 Records of decay-in-storage.

Records of disposal of licensed materials must be maintained for 3 years and must include the date of the disposal, the survey instrument used, the background radiation level, the radiation level measured at the surface of each waste container, and the name of the individual who performed the survey.

10 CFR 35.2204 Records of ^{99}Mo concentrations.

Records of ^{99}Mo concentration tests must be maintained for 3 years and must include, for each measured elution of ^{99m}Tc, the ratio of the measures expressed as μCi Mo/mCi Tc (kBq ^{99}Mo/MBq ^{99m}Tc), the time and date of the measurement, and the name of the individual who made the measurement.

9.12.2 Discussion of the Requirements

The required records are self-explanatory. Clear distinctions also must be made among the quantities entered on some of these records (e.g., total effective dose equivalent, shallow-dose equivalent, lens dose equivalent, deep-dose equivalent, or committed effective dose equivalent).

9.12.3 Suggested Procedures for Compliance

Licensees should be able to easily develop forms for each of the required records based on the information in this section. Each required record must be legible throughout the specified retention period. The licensee must maintain adequate safeguards against tampering with and loss of these records.

9.13 Reports

9.13.1 Pertinent Regulations

10 CFR 19.13 Notifications and reports to individuals. Radiation exposure data for an individual and the results of any measurements, analyses, and calculations of radioactive material deposited or retained in the body of an individual must be reported to the individual. Each worker must be advised annually of his or her dose.

10 CFR 20.2201 Reports of theft or loss of licensed material. Licensees must notify the NRC Operation Center by telephone (301-951-0550) within 30 days after the occurrence of any lost, stolen, or missing licensed material becomes known in a quantity greater than 10 times that specified in Appendix C to Part 20. Quantities for the common radionuclides used in diagnostic nuclear medicine are shown in Table 9.5.

Within 30 days after the telephone report, a written report must be made to the administrator of the appropriate NRC Regional Office, containing the following information: description of the licensed material involved, description of the circumstances under which the loss or theft occurred, statement of disposition or probable disposition of licensed material involved, exposures of individuals to radiations, actions that have been taken to recover the material, and procedures that have been adopted to ensure against a recurrence of the loss or theft. Names of individuals who may have received exposure to radiation must be stated in a separate section of the report.

10 CFR 20.2203 Reports of exposures, radiation levels, and concentrations of radioactive material exceeding the constraints or limits.

A report must be submitted to U.S. NRC, Document Control Desk, Washington, DC 20555, with a copy to the appropriate NRC Regional Office, within 30 days after learning of any of the following:

(1) Doses in excess of any of the following: occupational dose limits for adults or minors, limits for an embryo/fetus of a declared pregnant

Reports

Pertinent regulations:

10 CFR 19.13	Notifications and reports to individuals
10 CFR 20.2201	Reports of theft or loss of licensed material
10 CFR 20.2203	Reports of exposures, radiation levels, and concentrations of radioactive material exceeding the constraints or limits
10 CFR 20.2205	Reports of individuals exceeding dose limits
10 CFR 30.50	Reporting requirements
10 CFR 35.3045	Report and notification of a medical event
10 CFR 35.3047	Report and notification of a dose to an embryo/fetus or a nursing child
10 CFR 35.3067	Report of a leaking source

The complete text of these regulations can be accessed online through the NRC electronic reading room at www.nrc.gov.

TABLE 9.5
Quantities of Common Radionuclides to be Reported to NRC if Lost or Stolen

Radionuclide	Quantity (mCi)
^{18}F	10
^{57}Co (sealed source)	1
^{67}Ga	10
^{99m}Tc	10
^{111}In	1
^{123}I	1
^{131}I	0.01
^{133}Xe	10
^{137}Cs (sealed source)	0.1
^{201}Tl	10

*SI conversion factor: 1 mCi = 37 MBq.

worker, limits for an individual member of the public, or the as low as reasonably achievable constraints for air emissions; or

(2) Levels of radiation or concentrations of radioactive material in a restricted area in excess of any applicable limit or in an unrestricted area in excess of 10 times any applicable limit.

Each report must describe the extent of exposure of individuals to radioactive material, including, as appropriate: estimate of each individual's dose; levels of radiation and concentrations of radioactive material involved; cause of the elevated exposures, dose rates, or concentrations; and corrective steps taken to ensure against a recurrence. The report also must include a separate section for each occupationally overexposed individual containing his or her name, Social Security number, and date of birth.

10 CFR 20.2205 Reports of individuals exceeding dose limits.

When a licensee is required, pursuant to § 20.2203, to report to the Commission any exposure of an identified occupationally exposed individual or an identified member of the public to radioactive material, the licensee must also provide a copy of the report to the individual.

10 CFR 30.50 Reporting requirements.

Each licensee must notify the NRC as soon as possible but not later than 4 hours after the discovery of an event that prevents immediate protective actions necessary to avoid exposures to radioactive materials that could exceed regulatory limits (events may include fires, explosions, etc.).

Each licensee must notify the NRC within 24 hours after the discovery of any unplanned medical treatment of an individual with spreadable radioactive contamination on the individual's clothing or body.

Licensees must first make telephone notification to the NRC Operations Center (301-816-5100) with the following information: caller's name and call back number; description of the event; exact location of event; isotopes, quantities, and chemical and physical form of licensed material involved; and any personnel radiation exposure data available. A written report must be submitted within 30 days to the U.S. NRC, Document Control Desk, Washington, DC 20555, with a copy to the appropriate NRC Regional Office, and must include the following: description of event; exact location of event; isotopes, quantities, and chemical and physical form of licensed material involved; date and time of event; corrective actions taken; and extent of exposure of individuals to radioactive materials without identification of individuals by name.

10 CFR 35.3045 Report and notification of a medical event.

A licensee must report any event, except for an event resulting from patient intervention, in which the administration of licensed material results in:

(1) A dose that differs from prescribed dosage by >5 rem (0.05 Sv) effective dose equivalent (EDE), 50 rem (0.5 Sv) to an organ or tissue, or 50 rem (0.5 Sv) shallow-dose equivalent (SDE) to the skin; and the total dosage delivered differs from the prescribed dosage by 20% or more or falls outside the prescribed dosage range; or

(2) A dose >5 rem (0.05 Sv) EDE, 50 rem (0.5 Sv) to an organ or tissue, or 50 rem (0.5 Sv) SDE to the skin from any of the following: administration of the wrong radioactive drug, administration of a radioactive drug by a wrong route of administration, administration of dosage to the wrong individual or human research subject, or a leaking sealed source.

A licensee must report any event resulting from patient intervention or human research subject in which the administration of licensed material will result in unintended permanent functional damage to an organ or a physiological system, as determined by a physician. (Patient intervention means actions by the patient or human research subject, whether intentional or unintentional, such as dislodging or removing treatment devices or prematurely terminating the administration.)

Licensee must notify the NRC Operations Center by telephone (301-951-0550) no later than the next calendar day after discovery of the medical event. A written report must be submitted to the appropriate NRC Regional Office within 15 days and must include: licensee's name; name of prescribing physician; brief description of event; why event occurred; effect, if any, on individual(s) who received the administration; actions taken, if any, to prevent recurrence; and certification that licensee notified the individual (or responsible relative or guardian), and if not, why not. The report may not contain any information that could lead to identification of the individual. The licensee must also provide an annotated copy of the report to the referring physician no later than 15 days after the discovery of the event, with the name of the affected individual and his or her Social Security number or other identification number.

The licensee must provide notification of the event to the referring physician and also notify the involved individual no later than 24 hours after discovery of the event, unless the referring physician personally informs the licensee either that he or she will inform the individual or that, based on medical judgment, telling the individual would be harmful. The licensee is not required to notify the individual without first consulting the referring physician. If the referring physician or affected individual cannot be reached within 24 hours, the licensee must notify the individual as soon as possible thereafter (if necessary, notification may be made to responsible relative or guardian). The licensee may not delay any appropriate medical care for the individual. If a verbal notification is made, the licensee must inform the individual that a written description of the event can be obtained upon request.

Aside from notification, nothing in this requirement affects any rights or duties of licensees and physicians in relation to each other, to individuals affected by the medical event, or to that individual's responsible relatives or guardians.

10 CFR 35.3047 Report and notification of a dose to an embryo/fetus or a nursing child.

A licensee must report any dose to an embryo/fetus that is >5 rem (0.05 Sv) dose equivalent that is a result of an administration of byproduct material to a pregnant individual, unless the dose was specifically approved, in advance, by the authorized user.

A licensee must report any dose to a nursing child that is a result of an administration of byproduct material to a breast feeding woman that is > 5 rem (0.05 Sv) total effective dose equivalent or has resulted in unintended permanent functional damage to an organ or a physiological system of the child, as determined by a physician.

Regulatory Issues at a Glance: Reports

- Appropriate reports
- Notifications to individuals
- Theft or loss of licensed material
- Exposures, radiation levels, and radioactive concentrations exceeding limits
- Individuals exceeding dose limits
- 10 CFR 30.50 requirements
- Medical event
- Dose to embryo/fetus or nursing child
- Leaking source

Notification consists of first telephoning the NRC Operations Center no later than the next calendar day after discovery of the event, followed by a written report to the appropriate NRC Regional Office within 15 days that includes: licensee's name; name of prescribing physician; brief description of event; why event occurred; effect, if any, on embryo/fetus or nursing child; actions taken, if any, to prevent recurrence; and certification that licensee notified pregnant individual or mother (or responsible relative or guardian), and if not, why not. The report must not contain any information that could lead to identification of the individual or child. The licensee must also provide an annotated copy of the report to the referring physician no later than 15 days after the discovery of the event, with the name of the pregnant individual or the nursing child and his or her Social Security number or other identification number.

The licensee must provide notification of the event to the referring physician and also notify the pregnant individual or mother (both hereafter referred to as the mother), no later than 24 hours after discovery of the event, unless the referring physician personally informs the licensee either that he or she will inform the mother or that, based on medical judgment, telling the mother would be harmful. The licensee is not required to notify the mother without first consulting with the referring physician. If the referring physician or mother cannot be reached within 24 hours, the licensee must make the appropriate notifications as soon as possible thereafter (if necessary, notification may be made to a responsible relative or guardian). The licensee may not delay any appropriate medical care for the embryo/fetus or for the nursing child. If a verbal notification is made, the licensee must inform the mother that a written description of the event can be obtained upon request.

10 CFR 35.3067 Report of a leaking source.

Report must be filed within 5 days with the appropriate NRC Regional Office, with a copy to the Director, Office of Nuclear Material Safety and Safeguards, U.S. NRC, Washington, DC 20555-001, if a leak test reveals the presence of 0.005 μCi (185 Bq) or more of removable contamination and must include the model number and serial number if assigned, of the leaking source; the radionuclide and its estimated activity; the results of the test; the date of the test; and the action taken.

9.13.2 Discussion of the Requirements

Most of the required reports are self-explanatory. The incidents referred to in § 30.50 are unusual occurrences. In this requirement, the terms "unplanned medical treatment" and "spreadable radioactive contamination" are not defined. These appear to involve radiation accidents involving injuries and contamination unrelated to nuclear medicine; however, the treatment of such patients becomes an NRC issue.

9.13.3 Suggested Procedures for Compliance

Licensees should be able to easily develop forms for each of the required reports based on the information in this section. It is anticipated that the reporting of some of these events (e.g., medical events and unauthorized medical exposure of embryo/fetus) will be extremely rare occurrences. Permanent functional damage to an organ or a physiological system should never occur. Licensees should refer to the radiation doses received from common diagnostic nuclear medicine procedures listed in Chapter 2.

9.14 Safety Instruction for Workers

9.14.1 Pertinent Regulations

10 CFR 19.12 Instruction to workers.

All workers who are likely to receive an annual occupational dose in excess of 100 mrem (1 mSv) must be:

(1) Kept informed of the storage, transfer, or use of radioactive material;
(2) Instructed in radiation protection and the applicable NRC regulations;
(3) Instructed to report promptly any condition that may cause a violation of NRC regulations;
(4) Instructed in the appropriate response in the event of any unusual occurrence that may involve radiation exposure; and
(5) Advised that they may view their radiation exposure reports if they are issued dosimetry or have bioassay measurement taken pursuant to § 19.13. Workers likely to receive >100 mrem/y (1mSv/y) but not likely to receive 500 mrem/y (5 mSv/y) are not required to be issued dosimeters.

10 CFR 35.27 Supervision.

Licensees must:

(1) Instruct all supervised individuals in the licensee's written radiation protection procedures and all applicable regulations and license conditions; and
(2) Require that supervised individuals follow instructions of supervising authorized users (AU) for medical use of byproduct material, written radiation protection procedures established by licensee, and all applicable regulations and license conditions.

Licensees are responsible for the acts and omissions of the supervised individual.

Safety Instruction for Workers

Pertinent regulations:

10 CFR 19.12	Instruction to workers
10 CFR 35.27	Supervision

The complete text of these regulations can be accessed online through the NRC electronic reading room at www.nrc.gov.

9.14.2 Discussion of the Requirements

AUs and their supervised employees are most likely to receive doses >100 mrem (1 mSv) in a year. Essentially all diagnostic nuclear medicine licensees permit the receipt, possession, use, transfer, and preparation of byproduct material by an individual under the supervision of an AU (e.g., nuclear medicine technologist). All individuals who are likely to receive radiation doses >100 mrem (the dose limit for members of the public) must be instructed in radiation safety. There is neither a requirement to continually train these individuals nor a time interval specified for any necessary instruction. (This so-called "refresher training" is often performed as the result of a license condition).

It may be prudent to instruct certain individuals, even if they are not likely to receive 100 mrem (1 mSv) (e.g., housekeeping staff and security). For example, housekeeping staff could be informed of the nature of the licensed material and the meaning of the radiation symbol, instructed not to touch any licensed material, and told which areas are "off-limits." Providing this minimal instruction to ancillary staff may assist in controlling abnormal events, such as loss of radioactive material.

If radiation workers are likely to receive radiation doses that are <500 mrem (5 mSv), personnel monitoring of these individuals is not required (see section 9.2). Because a radiation worker is NOT a member of the public and has consented to work with radioactive materials, it is not reasonable (ALARA) to maintain their doses at 100 mrem (1 mSv), but rather 500 mrem (5 mSv). Recall that under § 35.75 the 500-mrem limit applies to the public as well if the exposure is from a released patient.

9.14.3 Suggested Procedures for Compliance

Safety instruction for professional staff (e.g., AU, radiation safety officer, nuclear medicine technologist) in diagnostic nuclear medicine may contain the following topics:

(1) Storage, transfer, and use of radioactive materials.
(2) Health protection problems associated with exposure to radiation and/or radioactive material.
(3) Precautions or procedures to minimize exposure.
(4) Purposes and functions of protective devices.
(5) Applicable NRC regulations and any license conditions.
(6) Licensee's written radiation protection procedures.
(7) Responsibility to report promptly any condition that may cause a violation of NRC regulations or an unnecessary radiation exposure.
(8) Appropriate response in the event of any unusual occurrence that may involve radiation exposure.
(9) Worker requests for radiation exposure reports.

For mobile diagnostic nuclear medicine service providers, safety instruction may contain applicable U.S. Department of Transportation regulations.

If staff and procedures have not changed in a given year, the instruction obviously should be minimized. New employees must receive appropriate safety instruction, but there is no requirement to continually train those supervised individuals who are already adequately trained. In this case, instruction should not involve review of procedures and basic radiation safety knowledge that the individual routinely uses and is familiar with but, instead, should be limited to topics with which the individual is not involved frequently. It would also be prudent to instruct, for example, veteran nuclear medicine technologists after significant changes in regulations, terms of the license, procedures, or type of licensed material used.

Although instruction is a Part 19 requirement for all individuals likely to receive a dose >100 mrem (1 mSv), these same individuals do not have to be monitored if their radiation dose is likely to be <500 mrem (5 mSv). If, based on historical personnel dosimetry data, individuals are not likely to receive 500 mrem, then the need for any continual safety instruction of

Regulatory Issues at a Glance: Safety Instruction for Workers

Instruction to workers
Supervised individuals

veteran workers (unless warranted by any significant changes noted previously) seems overly burdensome. In such circumstances, licensees should consider applying to the NRC for an exemption to this safety instruction requirement under § 19.31, because an exemption, if granted, will not result in undue hazard to life or property.

9.15 Audit Program

9.15.1 Pertinent Regulations

10 CFR 20.1101 Radiation protection programs.
Licensees must, at least annually, review the radiation protection program content and implementation.

10 CFR 20.2102 Records of radiation protection programs.
Licensees must maintain records of audits and other reviews of the radiation protection program content and implementation.

9.15.2 Discussion of the Requirements

Licensees must review and/or audit, on an annual basis, their radiation protection program's content, implementation, and effectiveness. This is important so that any violations or radiation safety concerns that may be identified can be corrected in a timely manner. Not all deficiencies need result in corrective actions as long as appropriate reasons can be given. These reviews may also indicate that certain procedures and/or requirements should be minimized or even eliminated. In such cases, licensees should appropriately alter their radiation protection policies and implementing procedures and/or apply to the NRC for an exemption from the applicable requirements in Parts 19, 20, 30, and 35 (as discussed in section 9.1).

Audit Program

Pertinent regulations:

10 CFR 20.1101	Radiation protection programs
10 CFR 20.2102	Records of radiation protection programs

The complete text of these regulations can be accessed online through the NRC electronic reading room at www.nrc.gov.

Regulatory Issues at a Glance: Audit Program

Review of radiation protection policies and implementing procedures

9.15.3 Suggested Procedures for Compliance

All aspects of the licensee's radiation protection program must be reviewed on an annual basis. The audit should be performed with the following three questions in mind:

(1) What can happen?
(2) How likely is it?
(3) What are the consequences?

Form 9.1 contains a list of the items to be checked and can be used for auditing the radiation protection program.

9.16. Mobile Diagnostic Nuclear Medicine Services (if applicable)

9.16.1 Pertinent Regulations

10 CFR 35.80 Provision of mobile medical service.
A licensee providing mobile medical service must:

(1) Obtain a letter signed by each client's management for which services are rendered that permits use of byproduct material at client's address and delineates authority and responsibility of licensee and client;
(2) Check instruments used to measure activity of unsealed byproduct material for proper function (at a minimum, perform constancy check) before medical use at each client's address or on each day of use, whichever is more frequent;

Mobile Diagnostic Nuclear Medicine Services

Pertinent regulations:

10 CFR 35.80	Provision of mobile medical service
10 CFR Part 71	Packaging and transportation of radioactive material

Department of Transportation regulations in 49 CFR Parts 170–189

(3) Check survey instruments for proper operation with dedicated check source before use at each client's address; and

(4) Before leaving client's address, survey all areas of use to ensure compliance with dose limits requirements in Part 20.

A mobile medical service may not have byproduct material delivered from the manufacturer or distributor to the client unless the client has a license allowing possession of the byproduct material. Byproduct material delivered to client must be received and handled in conformance with the client's license.

10 CFR Part 71 Packaging and Transportation of Radioactive Material
Various sections

Department of Transportation (DOT) regulations in 49 CFR Parts 170–189.

9.16.2 Discussion of the Requirements

A mobile medical service means the transportation of byproduct material to and its medical use at the client's address (§ 35.2). Mobile medical service licensees may transport licensed material and equipment into a client's building or may bring patients into the transport (e.g., van). In either case, the van should be located on the client's property that is under the client's control. In-van-imaging-only services may not be considered an NRC-licensed activity if byproduct material is not administered, possessed, or used. Most mobile diagnostic nuclear medicine services are self-contained (byproduct material, trained personnel, and the facility), providing an administration area, radioactive waste storage, trained personnel, radiation safety equipment (e.g., dose calibrator and survey instruments), and imaging equipment. A second type of mobile service provider (byproduct material and trained personnel) offers transportation to and use of the byproduct material within the client's facility.

In the NRC license application, the applicant must describe the type of mobile medical service to be provided. The base location(s) must also be specified, and multiple base locations may be requested (radioactive material must be delivered only to a facility licensed to receive the type of radioactive material ordered). The base facility may be located in a medical institution, noninstitutional medical practice, commercial facility, or mobile van.

9.16.3 Suggested Procedures for Compliance

In addition to the specific regulations given in § 35.80, the licensee also must comply with all applicable regulations for any diagnostic nuclear medicine facility (given elsewhere in this chapter). Additional training that includes all applicable DOT regulations should be provided.

Byproduct material will be delivered by a supplier to the base location or to the client's address if the client is licensed to receive the type of byproduct material ordered. Delivery of byproduct material to a van will be permitted only if occupied by authorized personnel. Byproduct material may be picked up, if necessary, from the supplier en route to client facilities. If radioactive waste is stored in vans, the vans must be properly secured and posted. Excreta from individuals undergoing medical diagnosis may be disposed of without regard to radioactivity if it is discharged into the sanitary sewerage system. However, collecting excreta from patients in a van restroom with a holding tank is not considered direct disposal into the sanitary sewerage system. If restroom facilities are provided in the van for patient use, the following additional radiation protection policies and implementing procedures should be added to the radiation protection program:

(1) Considerations of tank holding facility and location of tank in relation to members of the public and workers in the van (or driver);

(2) Procedures to assess the tank for possible leakage;

(3) Procedures to ensure that doses to occupational workers and members of the public will not exceed applicable limits and are maintained as low as reasonably achievable; and

(4) Procedures for emptying and disposing of contents of holding tank.

NRC licensees who want to conduct operations in Agreement States should contact that state's Radiation Control Program Office to clarify requirements and to determine whether mobile medical services are allowed within that Agreement State through reciprocity. Agreement State licensees that request reciprocity for activities conducted in non-Agreement States are subject to the general license provisions described in 10 CFR 150.20 *Recognition of Agreement State Licenses.*

This general license authorizes persons holding a specific license from an Agreement State in which the licensee maintains an office for directing the licensed activity and retaining radiation safety records to conduct the same activity in non-Agreement States if the specific license issued does not limit the authorized activity to specific locations or installations.

Regulatory Issues at a Glance: Mobile Diagnostic Nuclear Medicine Services

- Appropriately signed letter for each client
- Proper functioning of dose calibrator
- Proper operation of survey instruments
- Required surveys
- Byproduct material receipt
- Reciprocity
- Department of Transportation regulations
- In-van restroom facilities

FORM 9.1

Radiation Protection Program Audit

Date of review:______________ Date of last review:______________

Reviewer:______________________________________ Date:__________________
(Name and signature)

Management review:______________________________ Date:__________________
(Name and signature)

Audit History

1. Were previous audits conducted annually?
2. Were records of previous audits maintained?
3. Were any deficiencies identified during previous audits?
4. Were corrective actions taken?

Radiation Protection Program (General)

1. Radiation protection policies and implementing procedures in place?
2. Authority and responsibilities delineated?
3. Has management delegated authority to the radiation safety officer (RSO)?
4. Has the RSO agreed in writing to be responsible for program?
5. As low as reasonably achievable (ALARA) policy?
6. Any amendments requested?
7. Recent NRC or state inspection?
8. Any notices of violation, penalties, or orders and any licensee response?
9. Appropriate documentation provided to NRC before and/or after the following individuals started or stopped working: authorized user (AU), radiation safety officer (RSO), authorized nuclear pharmacist (ANP), or authorized medical physicist (AMP)?
10. If control of license was transferred or bankruptcy filed, was NRC prior consent obtained or notification made?

Training and Experience

1. Does AU meet NRC training requirements?
2. Does RSO meet NRC training requirements? (ANP and AMP meet NRC training requirements?)
3. Is RSO fulfilling all duties?
4. If RSO was changed, was license amended?
5. Recentness of training?

Occupational Dose Limits

1. Dose limits for adults maintained?
2. Dose limits for minors maintained?
3. Any declared pregnant workers?
   a. Dose limits for embryo/fetus maintained?
4. External dosimetry:
   a. Workers monitored properly, if required?
   b. Supplier approved by the National Voluntary Laboratory Accreditation Program?
   c. Dosimeters exchanged at required frequency?
5. Internal dosimetry:
   a. Workers monitored, if required?
6. Protective clothing worn?
7. Personnel routinely monitor their hands?
8. No eating/drinking/personal effects in use/storage areas?

Dose Limits for Members of the Public

1. Dose limits for public maintained?
2. Surveys performed, if required?
3. Air emissions to environment?

Minimization of Contamination/Spill Procedures

1. Facilities as described in license?
2. Has radioactive contamination and generation of waste been minimized?
3. Any spills requiring change in procedures?

Material Receipt and Accountability/Ordering, Receiving, and Opening Packages

1. Licensed material in storage secured from unauthorized removal or access?
2. Licensed material not in storage controlled and under constant surveillance?
3. Radionuclide, chemical form, quantity, and use as authorized?
4. Appropriate approval required to order licensed material?
5. Packages received and opened appropriately?

(continued)

Radiation Surveys and Calibration of Survey Instruments

1. Appropriate external dose rate and radioactive contamination (wipe) surveys performed?
2. Appropriate instruments used?
3. Instruments calibrated annually and after repairs?
4. Are personnel knowledgeable in instrument operation?

Caution Signs and Posting Requirements

1. All required documents or notices posted?
2. Caution signs adequately posted?
3. All areas in which radioactive materials storied or used appropriately posted?

Labeling Containers, Vials, and Syringes

1. Containers, vials, and syringes labeled properly?
2. Syringe and vial shields used?

Determining Patient Dosages

1. Each dosage determined and recorded before medical use?
2. Dose calibrator required?
   a. If not, is measurement of unit dosage made by decay correction, or, for other than unit dosage, is measurement made by combination of volumetric measurement and calculation? Any ^{99m}Tc radiopharmaceuticals administered with >0.15 μCi ^{99}Mo/mCi ^{99m}Tc (>0.15 kBq^{99}Mo/MBq ^{99m}Tc)?
   b. If required or used, are the following procedures in place?
      i. Calibration in accordance with nationally recognized standards or manufacturer's instructions?
      ii. Dose calibrator repaired or replaced as required?
      iii. If using a molybdenum/technetium generator, is first eluate after receipt tested for ^{99}Mo?
      iv. Any ^{99m}Tc radiopharmaceuticals administered with >0.15 μCi ^{99}Mo/mCi ^{99m}Tc (>0.15 kBq^{99}Mo/MBq ^{99m}Tc)?

Sealed Source Inventory and Leak Testing

1. Appropriate authorization for calibration, transmission, and reference sources?
2. Sealed sources inventoried?
3. Leak tests performed on sealed sources?

Waste Disposal and Decay-in-Storage

1. Radioactive waste disposed of in properly labeled receptacles?
2. Radioactive waste secured and area properly posted?
3. Proper disposal: decay-in-storage, procedures followed, labels removed/defaced?
4. Any improper/unauthorized disposals?
5. If used, are molybdenum/technetium generators disposed of properly?

Records/Reports

1. Appropriate records kept?
2. Appropriate reports written?

Safety Instruction for Workers

1. Is safety instruction being given to workers if needed?
2. Is the individual's understanding of current procedures and regulations adequate?

Mobile Diagnostic Nuclear Medicine Services (if applicable)

1. Dose calibrator checked for proper functioning at each client's address?
2. Survey instruments checked for proper operation before use at each client's address?
3. All areas of use surveyed before leaving client's address?
4. Appropriately signed letter for each client? Reciprocity?
5. Byproduct material received in accordance with the license? Training in U.S. Department of Transportation regulations?

Audit Findings

1. Summary of findings:
   a. Any appropriate program changes (any procedures identified that could be minimized or eliminated?
   b. Any exemptions from applicable requirements that should be requested)o?
2. Corrective and preventive actions:

10 License Application

10.1 Application Process and License Issuance

To apply for an NRC license in diagnostic nuclear medicine, an applicant must do the following (§ 35.12):

(1) File an original and one copy of NRC Form 313, Application for Material License, that includes the facility diagram, equipment, and training and experience qualifications of the radiation safety officer (RSO) and authorized user(s) (AU) (if applicable, also authorized medical physicists [AMPs] and authorized nuclear pharmacists [ANPs]); and

(2) Have applicant or licensee management sign the application.

The submission of written procedures to meet the requirements of the applicable regulations is not required as part of the license application process. However, the applicant must provide a commitment to "develop, document, and implement" these procedures as they will be examined during NRC inspections. The suggested procedures detailed in Chapter 9 can be used for this purpose. The applicant must also provide any other information requested by the NRC in its review of the application.

The NRC will issue a license for the medical use of byproduct material if (§ 35.18):

(1) The applicant has filed NRC Form 313, Application for Material License, in accordance with the instructions in § 35.12;

(2) The applicant has paid any applicable fee as provided in 10 CFR Part 170;

(3) The Commission finds the applicant equipped and committed to observe the required safety standards established for the protection of the public health and safety; and

(4) The applicant meets the requirements of 10 CFR Part 30.

The first step in filing for an NRC materials license is to complete NRC Form 313. The Form consists of 13 items; items 1–4, 12, and 13 can be completed on the form itself, whereas items 5–11 require supplementary pages. The following section explains and provides suggested responses, item by item, for the information requested on NRC Form 313 for diagnostic nuclear medicine facilities seeking a specific license of limited scope to use unsealed byproduct material prepared for medical use for imaging and localization studies (i.e., § 35.200 material).

At a Glance: Elements of License Application

Item 1.	License Action Type
Item 2.	Applicant's Name and Mailing Address
Item 3.	Address(es) Where Licensed Material Will Be Used
Item 4.	Contact Person
Item 5.	Radioactive Material
Item 6.	Purpose(s) for Use of Licensed Material
Item 7.	Individual(s) Responsible for Radiation Safety Program and Their Training and Experience
Item 8.	Safety Instruction for Individuals Working in Restricted Areas
Item 9.	Facilities and Equipment
Item 10.	Radiation Protection Program
Item 11.	Waste Management
Item 12.	Fees
Item 13.	Certification

10.1.1 Item 1. License Action Type

Check the box for a new license (for amendments or renewals, see Chapter 11).

10.1.2 Item 2. Applicant's Name and Mailing Address

The legal name of the applicant's facility must be given. This is the entity that has direct control over use of the radioactive material. Nuclear medicine divisions or departments within hospitals may not be listed. The mailing address also must be provided.

Note: The NRC must be notified before control of the license is transferred, whenever bankruptcy proceedings are initiated, or when a licensee decides to permanently cease licensed activities:

Notification of Transfer of Control

Licensees must provide full information and obtain NRC's written consent before transferring control of the license (§ 30.34(b)). A simple name change that does not involve transfer of control of the license or mailing address change only requires written notification with NRC no later than 30 days after the date of the change.

Notification of Bankruptcy Proceedings

Immediately (i.e., within 24 hours) after the filing of a bankruptcy petition, a licensee must notify the NRC. This is because the NRC wants to ensure that there will be no public health and safety concerns. The licensee remains responsible for compliance with all regulatory requirements.

Termination of Activities/License Termination

For diagnostic nuclear medicine licenses, license termination does not require much, because the total inventory of licensed material will not exceed regulatory limits and because the half-lives of the unsealed byproduct materials are so short. The NRC must be notified, in writing, within 60 days, when the license has expired or a decision has been made to permanently cease licensed activities at the entire site. Licensees must certify the disposition of licensed materials and that the facility is not contaminated to facilitate decommissioning (i.e., release of the site for unrestricted use). For the interested reader, Subpart E to 10 CFR Part 20 describes the radiological criteria for license termination.

10.1.3 Item 3. Address(es) Where Licensed Material Will Be Used

The address should specify a street address, not a post office box, because the address must be sufficient to allow NRC inspectors to find the facility location.

If applying for a license for a mobile diagnostic nuclear medicine service, the type of mobile medical service to be provided must be described (see section 9.16). The base location(s) also must be specified. Multiple base locations may be requested. (Radioactive material must be delivered only to a facility licensed to receive the type of radioactive material ordered.) The base facility may be located in a medical institution, noninstitutional medical practice, commercial facility, or mobile van. When the base facility is the mobile van, specify whether a permanent structure is used for byproduct material storage. If not, provide the following:

(1) Secured off-street parking under licensee control;
(2) Secured storage facilities (for byproduct material and radioactive waste) available if the van is disabled; and
(3) Byproduct material delivered (if necessary) directly to the van only if the van is occupied by licensee personnel at time of delivery.

If the base facility is located in a residential area, provide the following:

(1) Justification of need for private residence, rather than commercial, location;
(2) Documentation of agreement between residence owner and licensee;
(3) Description of program demonstrating compliance with 10 CFR 20.1301, *Dose limits for individual members of the public;* and
(4) Verification that restricted areas do not contain residential quarters.

Note: Applicants requesting a mobile service license should contact all Agreement States, if any, in which they plan to conduct operations to clarify requirements and to determine whether mobile medical services are allowed within that Agreement State through reciprocity (see section 9.16).

10.1.4 Item 4. Contact Person

A person knowledgeable about the application and the facility should be listed as the contact person (typically the proposed RSO), because the NRC will contact this individual if there are questions about the application. The telephone number of this individual also must be included.

10.1.5 Item 5. Radioactive Material

The form specifies: a. element and mass number; b. chemical and/or physical form; and c. maximum amount that will be possessed at any one time. Because this is an application for a specific license of limited scope for the use of § 35.200 material, the applicant should provide the following information:

a. Any byproduct material included in 10 CFR 35.200 (or 10 CFR 35.100, if applicable);

b. Any; and

c. As needed.

10.1.6 Item 6. Purpose(s) for Use of Licensed Material

The applicant can define the purposes of use by providing the statement, "Any imaging and localization procedure approved in 10 CFR 35.200" (or "Any uptake, dilution, and excretion procedure approved in 10 CFR 35.100," if applicable).

10.1.7 Item 7. Individual(s) Responsible for Radiation Safety Program and Their Training and Experience

NRC requires that an applicant be qualified by training and experience to use licensed materials for the purposes requested in such a manner as to protect health and minimize danger to life or property. For diagnostic nuclear medicine licensees, the personnel who typically have a role in the radiation protection program are the RSO and the AU physician(s). Their training and experience (see Chapter 8) must be documented in the license application (if ANPs and/or AMPs are involved, their training and experience must also be provided). NRC Form313a *Training and Experience and Preceptor Statement* may be used for this purpose.

Radiation Safety Officer (RSO)

Applicants must provide the name of the proposed RSO and his or her credentials demonstrating adequate training and experience as discussed in Chapter 8. In addition, the applicant should supply documentation indicating that management has delegated the authority for the day-to-day oversight of the radiation protection program to the RSO and that the RSO has agreed in writing to be responsible for implementing the radiation protection program.

Authorized Users (AUs)

Applicants must provide the name of the proposed AU(s) and their credentials demonstrating adequate training and experience in the use requested as discussed in Chapter 8.

10.1.8 Item 8. Safety Instruction for Individuals Working in Restricted Areas

Individuals working in the vicinity of licensed material must have adequate safety instruction as described in section 9.14. For mobile medical service providers, instruction also must include applicable DOT regulations. Licensees must have written policies and procedures in place; however, no response is necessary on the license application.

10.1.9 Item 9. Facilities and Equipment

The facilities and equipment must be adequate to protect health and minimize danger to life or property (§ 30.33(a)(2)). According to § 35.12, the application must include a diagram of the facility and describe the equipment necessary for the radiation protection program.

If applying for a license for a mobile diagnostic nuclear medicine service, the applicant must submit a diagram of the base facility; if more than one base facility, a diagram is necessary for each.

Facility Diagram

Applicants must submit a diagram that includes all rooms or areas in the facility. This diagram should indicate the principal use of each room or area. Restricted areas would include those areas in which byproduct material will be received, prepared, used, administered, and stored (e.g., hot lab, patient imaging rooms, and thyroid uptake room). Unrestricted or controlled areas would include the reception area, file room, waiting room, offices, hallways, and bathrooms. Any necessary shielding used and the location of additional radiation safety equipment (e.g., fume hood, room ventilation, xenon traps, and dose calibrator; see section 9.9 for the necessity of a dose calibrator) should be indicated on the diagram.

Equipment

Applicants should provide a list and description of all equipment (including the instrument type, sensitivity, and range for each type of radiation detected) that will be used for radiation protection.

Typically, diagnostic nuclear medicine licenses will need:

(1) Survey meters, typically a Geiger-Mueller or sodium iodide probes; they can be portable or fixed in a location, such as the hot lab (to be

used for ambient radiation surveys and personnel monitoring); if only one survey instrument will be used, licensee should describe procedures that will ensure access to a survey instrument when their instrument is being calibrated or repaired. If more than one survey instrument will be used, applicants should state that they will maintain at least one instrument at all times in order to make it clear that they are not committing to having all meters on the premises at all times; and

(2) NaI(Tl) well scintillation counter or other appropriate instrument used for assaying removable radioactive contamination; necessary for wipe testing of packages, sealed sources, and areas where unsealed byproduct material is prepared, administered or stored).

The applicant must also provide a statement, such as "We have developed and will document and implement written calibration procedures for survey meters and the NaI(Tl) well scintillation counter or other instrument in accordance with the applicable regulations." The following statement should also be included: "We reserve the right to upgrade our survey instruments as necessary, as long as they are adequate to measure the type and level of radiation for which they are used."

In addition, licensees using a dose calibrator (see section 9.9 for necessity of dose calibrator) should provide a statement, such as "We have developed and will document and implement written calibration procedures for the dose calibrator in accordance with nationally recognized standards or the manufacturer's instructions."

10.1.10 Item 10. Radiation Protection Program

The radiation protection program has been described in Chapter 9, along with suggested written radiation protection policies and implementing procedures to ensure compliance with all applicable NRC regulations. Applicants should provide a statement, such as "We have developed and will document and implement written procedures for a radiation protection program that will ensure compliance with all applicable NRC regulations and the security and safe use of unsealed byproduct material in diagnostic nuclear medicine. The program addresses training and experience requirements for the RSO and AU(s) (and ANP or AMP, if applicable), the safe use of unsealed licensed material, and each of the following:

(1) Occupational dose limits;
(2) Dose limits for members of the public;
(3) Minimization of contamination/spill procedures;
(4) Material receipt and accountability/ordering, receiving, and opening packages;
(5) Radiation surveys and calibration of survey instruments;
(6) Caution signs and posting requirements;
(7) Labeling containers, vials, and syringes;
(8) Determining patient dosages;
(9) Sealed source inventory and leak testing;
(10) Waste disposal and decay-in-storage;
(11) Records;
(12) Reports;
(13) Safety instruction for workers;
(14) Audit program; and
(15) Mobile diagnostic nuclear medicine services (if applicable)."

10.11.11 Item 11. Waste Management

Licensed materials must be disposed of in accordance with NRC requirements; these have been described along with suggested procedures in section 9.11. Applicants should provide a statement, such as "We have developed and will document and implement written waste disposal procedures in accordance with the applicable regulations."

For mobile medical service providers, if the van has restroom facilities in the van for patient use, the following information must be submitted for NRC review:

(1) Description of tank holding facility and location of tank in relation to members of the public and workers in the van (or driver) along with a description of procedures to assess the tank for possible leakage;
(2) Description of procedures to ensure doses to occupational workers and members of the public will not exceed applicable limits and are maintained as low as reasonably achievable; and

(3) Description of procedures for emptying and disposing of contents of holding tank.

10.1.12 Item 12. Fees

Enter the appropriate fee category from 10 CFR 170.31. For specific licenses of limited scope, this is category 7 for medical licenses, subcategory C. The fee amount must be enclosed with the application. For broad scope licenses, this is category 7, subcategory B.

10.1.13 Item 13. Certification

Typically, a representative of the legal entity filing the application should sign and date the application. This individual must be authorized to make binding commitments and to sign official documents on behalf of the applicant. An application for licensing a medical facility must be signed by the applicant's management, because, as previously discussed, signing the application acknowledges management's commitment and responsibilities for the radiation protection program.

Note: It is a criminal offense to make a willful false statement or representation on this application or any other correspondence with the NRC (18 U.S.C. 1001).

11

License Amendments and/or Renewals

It is the licensee's obligation to keep the license current. If any of the information provided in the original license application needs to be modified or changed by the licensee, an application for a license amendment should be submitted (§ 30.34 describes the terms and conditions of licenses). To request a license amendment or renewal from the NRC (§ 35.12), a diagnostic nuclear medicine licensee must submit an original and one copy of either NRC Form 313, *Application for Material License,* or a letter requesting the amendment or renewal (the license number should also be provided). A specific license of limited scope licensee must apply for and receive a license amendment before (§ 35.13):

(1) Receiving, preparing, or using byproduct material for a type of use that is permitted under Part 35 but that is not authorized on the license;

(2) Permitting anyone to work as an authorized user (AU), authorized medical physicist (AMP), or authorized nuclear physician (ANP), except those individuals who meet the board certification and recent training requirements in Part 35 or individuals who are recognized as AUs by the Commission or Agreement States*;

(3) Changing radiation safety officers (RSOs) (except when temporary RSOs);

(4) Receiving byproduct material in excess of the amount or in a different form, or receiving a different radionuclide than is authorized on the license; and

(5) Changing the address of use identified in the application or on the license.

All requests for license amendments or renewals must be approved in writing by the licensee's management.

According to § 35.14, a limited scope licensee must provide the necessary documentation (copy of board certification or license permit showing AU status) to the NRC no later than 30 days after it permits additional individuals to work as AUs*. Licensees must also notify the NRC by letter no later than 30 days after:

(1) An AU (or ANP or AMP) permanently discontinues performance of duties under the license or has a name change*;

(2) A RSO permanently discontinues performance of duties under the license or has a name change;

(3) The licensee's mailing address changes;

(4) The licensee's name changes, but the name change dose not constitute a transfer of control of the license; or

(5) The licensee has added to or changed the areas of use identified in the application or on the license where byproduct material is used in accordance with either § 35.100 or § 35.200*.

** Diagnostic nuclear medicine facilities in medical institutions with a specific license of broad scope are exempted from these provisions, and therefore are not required to obtain a license amendment or notify the NRC in these cases.*

Guide for Radiopharmaceutical Therapy

12 Introduction to Radiopharmaceutical Therapy

12.1 Background

This section of the book was developed to provide guidance to radiopharmaceutical therapy applicants and/or licensees in the implementation of the U.S. Nuclear Regulatory Commission's (NRC's) newly revised 10 CFR Part 35, *Medical Use of Byproduct Material.* This guidance is aimed at all licensees using unsealed byproduct material for which a written directive (i.e., a written order for the administration of byproduct material to a specific patient or human research subject) is required.

In 2002, the Society of Nuclear Medicine (SNM) and the American College of Nuclear Physicians (ACNP) published the *Guide for Diagnostic Nuclear Medicine* as an alternative to NRC licensing guidance, for implementation of the revised Part 35 regulations applicable to the practice of diagnostic nuclear medicine. The SNM/ACNP worked collaboratively with the NRC to develop this guide, and it has been licensed by the NRC for distribution to the medical community via the NRC Web site. The NRC has stated that the SNM/ACNP *Guide for Diagnostic Nuclear Medicine* "provides information that may be useful to nuclear medicine professionals in understanding the applicability of NRC requirements to the medical use of byproduct material in diagnostic settings and provides measures that practitioners may use to facilitate implementation of the revised rule." This guide now appears as Chapters 1–11 (pp. 1–73) of this book.

12.2 Scope of this Report

Additional guidance is necessary for the use of unsealed byproduct material in radiopharmaceutical therapy. The radiation protection policies and implementing procedures suggested in this book are an alternative to those given in NRC licensing guidance (NUREG-1556, Volume 9, *Consolidated Guidance About Material Licenses: Program-Specific Guidance About Medical Use Licenses.* Washington, DC: NRC; 2002). These policies and procedures were developed based on NRC regulations. They may not apply to licensed facilities in Agreement States. The NRC allows applicants and licensees to develop their own procedures rather than adopt the model procedures published as appendices to the NUREG. This material was designed to meet the needs of radiopharmaceutical therapy practitioners and serves as a companion to the material in Chapters 1–11 of this book. Together, these documents provide a comprehensive guide for diagnostic nuclear medicine and radiopharmaceutical therapy licensees in the medical use of unsealed byproduct materials.

13 The Practice of Radiopharmaceutical Therapy

The use of unsealed byproduct material in radiopharmaceutical therapy involves administering a radionuclide therapy agent to treat (including treatment as palliation) a specific disease. The most common use of unsealed byproduct material for therapy is the treatment of hyperthyroidism with Na ^{131}I. Other therapeutic procedures include ablation of thyroid cancer and its metastases, treatment of bone metastases in cancer patients, radioimmunotherapy of non-Hodgkin's lymphoma, treatment of malignant effusions, treatment of polycythemia vera and leukemia, and radiation synovectomy in patients with rheumatoid arthritis. Other radioimmunotherapy agents are likely to be added for routine cancer treatment in the near future.

The radionuclides used most often in therapeutic radiopharmaceuticals are ^{131}I, ^{153}Sm, ^{89}Sr, ^{90}Y, and ^{32}P. The most common therapeutic radionuclide procedures using these radiopharmaceuticals and their typical administered activities are shown in Table 13.1.

TABLE 13.1
Most Common Radiopharmaceutical Therapy Procedures

Radionuclide	Administered agent	Indication	Activities (mCi)
^{32}P	Phosphate	Polycythemia vera	4
	Chromic phosphate	Neoplastic effusions and Radiation synovectomy	3–5
^{89}Sr	Chloride	Bone pain	4
^{90}Y	Ibritumomab tiuxetan	Non-Hodgkin's lymphoma	32 (maximum)
^{131}I	Sodium iodide	Hyperthyroidism	10–30
	Sodium iodide	Thyroid cancer	100–400
	Tositumomab	Non-Hodgkin's lymphoma	85 (~average)
^{153}Sm	EDTMP	Bone pain	70

EDTMP = ethylenediamine tetramethylenephosphonic acid.

14

Revised Part 35 Requirements Applicable to Radiopharmaceutical Therapy Procedures

The revised 10 CFR Part 35 does not use or define the term "radiopharmaceutical therapy." Medical uses are categorized according to the written directive (i.e., a written order for the administration of byproduct material to a specific patient or human research subject) requirement (§ 35.40 and § 35.41) and physical form of byproduct material (unsealed material or sealed sources). Written directives are required for the administration of (1) Na ^{131}I in amounts >30 μCi (1.11 MBq), and (2) a therapeutic dosage of any other radiopharmaceutical.

Radiopharmaceutical therapy procedures are understood to be described or referenced in Subpart E, *Unsealed Byproduct Material—Written Directive Required,* specifically in Section 10 CFR 35.300, *Use of unsealed byproduct material for which a written directive is required.*

The following guide is applicable for all licensees using § 35.300 materials. In addition to the requirements for diagnostic nuclear medicine licensees detailed previously in this volume, licensees performing radionuclide therapy also must have specified training and experience, use written directives, and perform additional radiation surveys and may be required to institute a bioassay program.

14.1 Part 35 Subparts

The revised Part 35 rule is organized into Subparts A though N. The requirements for diagnostic and therapeutic medicine are intermingled. As a first step in making these requirements more user friendly, they were reviewed, and only those requirements applicable to diagnostic nuclear medicine were presented in the the first part of this book. Additional requirements for the use of § 35.300 materials in radiopharmaceutical therapy are shown in the following list. These requirements will be covered in Chapters 15 and 16.

Subpart A General Information

35.15 Exemptions regarding Type A specific licenses of broad scope.

Subpart B General Administrative Requirements

35.40 Written directives.

35.41 Procedures for administrations requiring a written directive.

Subpart C General Technical Requirements

35.70 Surveys of ambient radiation exposure rate.

35.75 Release of individuals containing unsealed byproduct material or implants containing byproduct material.

Subpart E Unsealed Byproduct Material—Written Directive Required

35.300 Use of unsealed byproduct material for which a written directive is required.

35.310 Safety instruction.

35.315 Safety precautions.

35.390 Training for use of unsealed byproduct material for which a written directive is required.

35.392 Training for the oral administration of Na ^{131}I requiring a written directive in quantities ≤33 mCi (1.22 GBq)

35.394 Training for the oral administration of Na ^{131}I requiring a written directive in quantities ≤33 mCi (1.22 GBq)

Subpart J Training and Experience Requirements (retained for 2-year period)

35.930 Training for therapeutic use of unsealed byproduct material.

35.932 Training for treatment of hyperthyroidism.

35.934 Training for treatment of thyroid carcinoma.

Subpart L Records

35.2040 Records of written directives.

35.2041 Records for procedures for administrations requiring a written directive.

35.2070 Records of surveys for ambient radiation exposure rate.

35.2075 Records of the release of individuals containing unsealed byproduct material or implants containing byproduct material.

35.2310 Records of safety instruction.

Subpart M Reports

35.3045 Report and notification of a medical event.

35.3047 Report and notification of a dose to an embryo/fetus or a nursing child.

15

Training and Experience Requirements for Radiopharmaceutical Therapy Procedures

It is important to the radiation safety of workers and the public, including patients, to designate certain individuals who have adequate training and experience in radiation safety principles as applied to radiopharmaceutical therapy. This reduces unnecessary radiation exposure. Training and experience requirements to demonstrate sufficient knowledge and skills in radiation protection practices and procedures are essential for identifying individuals who may be recognized as:

(1) Authorized user physicians (AUs);
(2) Radiation safety officers (RSOs);
(3) Authorized nuclear pharmacists (ANPs); and
(4) Authorized medical physicists (AMPs).

The high level of protection afforded to patients, workers, and the public by the practice of radiopharmaceutical therapy is in part the result of the training and experience of these authorized individuals. Usually, these authorized individuals supervise other workers who are involved in medical use. They must direct these supervised individuals to ensure that unsealed byproduct material is handled safely. Radiopharmaceutical therapy procedures are usually performed in a nuclear medicine department, where nuclear medicine technologists and/or medical physicists may be involved, or in a radiation oncology department, where medical dosimetrists and/or medical physicists may participate in the administration of the radiopharmaceutical. However, no Nuclear Regulatory Commission (NRC) requirements specify their training and experience.

The NRC requires that an applicant/licensee be "qualified by training and experience to use licensed materials for the purposes requested in such a manner as to protect health and minimize danger to life or property" (§ 30.33). Therapeutic radionuclide purposes are the use of unsealed byproduct material for which a written directive is required, and these uses are covered by 10 CFR 35.300. Almost all licensees perform the studies in 10 CFR 35.300 and may use *any* unsealed byproduct material requiring a written directive prepared for medical use that is:

(1) Obtained from a manufacturer or preparer that is appropriately licensed by NRC or equivalent Agreement State requirements;
(2) Prepared by an ANP, a physician who is an AU and who meets the requirements in § 35.290, § 35.390, or, before October 24, 2004, § 35.290, or an individual under the supervision of either as specified in § 35.27;
(3) Obtained from and prepared by an NRC or Agreement State licensee for use in research in accordance with an Investigational New Drug (IND) protocol accepted by the U.S. Food and Drug Administration (FDA); or
(4) Prepared by a licensee for use in research in accordance with an IND protocol accepted by the FDA.

The NRC also has specific training and experience requirements for AUs whose practices are limited to the oral administration of Na ^{131}I, requiring a written directive in quantities ≤ 33 mCi (1.22 GBq), pursuant to § 35.392, or in quantities > 33 mCi (1.22 GBq), pursuant to § 35.394. Because the practice of radiopharmaceutical therapy, utilizing unsealed sources for which a written directive is needed, is not limited to these studies, the interested reader is referred to these latter pertinent regulations in 10 CFR Part 35.

The NRC training and experience requirements for AUs involved with § 35.300 materials and procedures are detailed here. NRC training and experience for RSOs are detailed in Chapter 8 and will not be reproduced here. Because most licensed facilities do not employ ANPs or AMPs, training and experience requirements for these individuals are not included. The interested reader is referred to the pertinent regulations (ANP: § 35.55, § 35.57, § 35.59, § 35.980, § 35.981; AMP: § 35.51, § 35.57, § 35.59, § 35.961).

15.1 Revised Requirements

The training and experience requirements in the revised Part 35 rule require that AUs meet either of the following two criteria:

(1) Certification by a medical specialty board whose certification process includes stated requirements and whose certification has been recognized by the NRC or an Agreement State; or

Completion of specified hours of didactic training and work experience under an AU; and

(2) Written certification signed by a preceptor AU.

Previously, AUs were required to be either certified by certain recognized specialty boards or obtain the requisite training and experience without written certification by a preceptor. As of April 2003, with the exception of the Certification Board of Nuclear Cardiology, no certifying boards are recognized by the NRC. The revised rule therefore includes a 2-year transition period for training and experience requirements. During this time the current or revised requirements may be used. According to 10 CFR Part 35.10, before October 25, 2004, a licensee can satisfy the requirements for AU status by complying with either:

(1) The appropriate training requirements in subpart J (§ 35.930); or

(2) The appropriate training requirements in § 35.390 (and/or § 35.57, § 35.59).

Subpart J of Part 35 has been retained for a 2-year period.

Note: As a result of concerns expressed by the NRC Advisory Committee on the Medical Uses of Isotopes, the Commission on February 12, 2003, directed the staff to prepare a proposed rule to modify the training and experience requirements.

15.1.1 Authorized User Physician

10 CFR 35.390 Training for use of unsealed byproduct material for which a written directive is required.

To become an AU of unsealed byproduct material for the uses authorized under § 35.300 a physician must meet one of the following criteria (except as provided in § 35.57):

(1) Certification by a medical specialty board whose certification process includes all of the requirements in item 2 and whose certification has been recognized by the Commission or an Agreement State.

(2) Completion of 700 hours of training and experience including all of the following:
  a. Classroom and laboratory training in:
    i. Radiation physics and instrumentation;
    ii. Radiation protection;
    iii. Mathematics pertaining to use and measurement of radioactivity;
    iv. Chemistry of byproduct material for medical use; and
    v. Radiation biology.
  b. Work experience under supervision of an AU who meets requirements in § 35.390 (*Note:* A supervising AU who is not board certified must have experience in administering dosages in the same dosage category or categories as the individual requesting AU status) or equivalent Agreement State requirements, involving:
    i. Ordering, receiving, and unpacking radioactive materials safely and performing related radiation surveys;
    ii. Calibrating instruments used to determine the activity of dosages and performing checks for proper operation of survey meters;
    iii. Calculating, measuring, and safely preparing patient or human research subject dosages;
    iv. Using administrative controls to prevent medical events involving use of unsealed byproduct material;
    v. Using procedures to safely contain spilled byproduct material and using proper decontamination procedures;
    vi. Eluting generator systems, measuring and testing the eluate for radionuclidic purity, and processing eluate with reagent kits to prepare labeled radioactive drugs; and

vii. Administering dosages of radioactive drugs to patients or human research subjects involving a minimum of three cases in each of the following categories for which the individual is requesting AU status:

1. Oral administration of ≤33 mCi (1.22 GBq) Na ^{131}I.
2. Oral administration of >33 mCi (1.22 GBq) Na ^{131}I (experience with three cases in this category also satisfies the requirement in category 1);
3. Parenteral administration of any beta emitter or a photon-emitting radionuclide with a photon energy <150 keV; and/or
4. Parenteral administration of any other radionuclide.

c. Obtained written certification, signed by a preceptor AU who meets requirements in § 35.390 or equivalent Agreement State requirements, that the individual has satisfactorily completed the requirements in 2a and 2b and has achieved a level of competency sufficient to function independently as an AU for the medical uses authorized under § 35.300.

Note: A preceptor AU who is not board certified must have experience in administering dosages in the same dosage category or categories (i.e., 2b(vii)(1–4)) as the individual requesting AU status.

10 CFR 35.930 Training for therapeutic use of unsealed byproduct material. (Subpart J; retained for 2 years)

To become an AU of radiopharmaceuticals in § 35.300, a physician must meet one of the following criteria (except as provided in § 35.57):

(1) Certification by any of the following:

a. The American Board of Nuclear Medicine;
b. The American Board of Radiology in radiology, therapeutic radiology, or radiation oncology;
c. The Royal College of Physicians and Surgeons of Canada in nuclear medicine; or
d. The American Osteopathic Board of Radiology after 1984.

(2) Completion of training and experience, including all of the following:

a. 80 hours of classroom and laboratory training in:
   i. Radiation physics and instrumentation;
   ii. Radiation protection;
   iii. Mathematics pertaining to use and measurement of radioactivity; and
   iv. Radiation biology.
b. Supervised clinical experience under supervision of AU at a medical institution that includes:
   i. Use of ^{131}I for diagnosis of thyroid function and the treatment of hyperthyroidism or cardiac dysfunction in 10 individuals; and
   ii. Use of ^{131}I for treatment of thyroid carcinoma in three individuals.

10 CFR 35.57 Training for experienced radiation safety officer, teletherapy or medical physicist, authorized user, and nuclear pharmacist.

Physicians identified as AUs for the medical use of byproduct material on a license issued by the Commission or Agreement State, a permit issued by a Commission master material licensee, a permit issued by a Commission or Agreement State broad scope licensee, or a permit issued by a Commission master material license broad scope permittee before October 24, 2002, who perform only those medical uses for which they were authorized on that date, need not comply with the training requirements of § 35.390.

10 CFR 35.59 Recentness of training.

The training and experience specified in § 35.390 and § 35.930 must have been obtained within the 7 years preceding the date of application, or the individual must have had related continuing education and experience since the required training and experience were completed.

16

Radiation Protection Program

A radiation protection program for diagnostic applications has been detailed in Chapter 9 of this volume, and most of these recommendations apply as well to practitioners involved in therapeutic medical uses of unsealed byproduct materials (utilizing unsealed sources for which a written directive is needed). Areas covered in Chapter 9 of the diagnostic guide are:

(1) Radiation protection program (general);
(2) Occupational dose limits;
(3) Dose limits for members of the public;
(4) Minimization of contamination/spill procedures;
(5) Material receipt and accountability/ordering, receiving, and opening packages;
(6) Radiation surveys and calibration of survey instruments;
(7) Caution signs and posting requirements;
(8) Labeling containers, vials, and syringes;
(9) Determining patient dosages;
(10) Sealed source inventory and leak testing;
(11) Waste disposal and decay-in-storage;
(12) Records;
(13) Reports;
(14) Safety instruction for workers;
(15) Audit program; and
(16) Mobile diagnostic nuclear medicine services.

Additional guidance is necessary for radiopharmaceutical therapy practitioners. Some of the 16 areas are expanded, and additional areas (written directives, release of individuals containing unsealed byproduct material, and safety procedures for treatment when patients are hospitalized) are given to provide:

(1) All pertinent Nuclear Regulatory Commission (NRC) requirements for the medical use of byproduct material in the practice of radiopharmaceutical therapy (utilizing unsealed sources for which a written directive is needed). These have been summarized in the interest of space; licensees should read the actual regulations. It should be noted that these are NRC regulations and, as such, may not apply in Agreement States. Practitioners in Agreement States must contact their respective rulemaking bodies.
(2) A discussion of the requirements; and
(3) Suggested procedures for compliance.

Note: Licensees will need to combine this chapter and Chapter 9 for a comprehensive radiation protection program.

16.1 Occupational Dose Limits

16.1.1 Pertinent Regulations

10 CFR 20.1202 Compliance with requirements for summation of external and internal doses.

If a licensee is required to monitor workers for both external and internal radiation dose under § 20.1502, the licensee must demonstrate compliance with the annual occupational dose limits by summing both contributions.

10 CFR 20.1204 Determination of internal exposure.

If a licensee is required to measure internal dose under § 20.1502 to demonstrate compliance with occupational dose limits, the licensee must take suitable and timely measurements of:

(1) Concentrations of radioactive materials in air in work areas;
(2) Quantities of radionuclides in the body;
(3) Quantities of radionuclides excreted from the body; or
(4) Combinations of these measurements.

10 CFR 20.1502(b) Conditions requiring individual monitoring of internal occupational dose.

Licensees must monitor the occupational intake of radioactive material and assess the committed effective dose equivalent (CEDE) to all of the following individuals:

(1) Adults likely to receive an annual intake >10% of the applicable annual limit on intake (ALI);
(2) Minors likely to receive an annual CEDE >0.1 rem (1 mSv); and
(3) Declared pregnant women (i.e., women who have voluntarily informed the licensee, in writing, of their pregnancy and the estimated date of conception) likely to receive a CEDE >0.1 rem (1 mSv) during the entire pregnancy.

16.1.2 Discussion of the Requirements

Radiation workers can receive radiation doses from two distinct sources: external exposure and internal intake. The total effective dose equivalent (TEDE) concept makes it possible to combine these dose components in assessing the overall risk to the health of an individual. The TEDE is equal to the sum of the deep-dose equivalent (DDE; from external exposures) and the CEDE (from internal exposures). These two sources of radiation dose also must be considered in demonstrating compliance with the annual dose limit for any individual organ or tissue, known as the total organ dose equivalent (TODE). The TODE is equal to the sum of the committed dose equivalent (CDE) (from intakes) and the DDE (from external radiation sources).

Licensees often decide to monitor all workers who are likely to be exposed to radioactive materials, regardless of the magnitude of exposure. However, personnel monitoring devices for measurement of external dose are required only for those workers who are likely to receive exposures in excess of the specified threshold of 500 mrem (5 mSv) from external radiation sources. Likewise, licensees are also required to monitor the occupational intakes of only those workers who are likely to exceed 10% of the specific ALI or CEDE limit. An intake of activity can occur by ingestion, inhalation, or skin absorption. The likelihood of internal intake by ingestion or inhalation depends on the radionuclide and its chemical and physical form.

If it can be demonstrated by air sampling or calculations that adult radiation workers are not likely to receive an annual intake >10% of an ALI (i.e., a CEDE per year dose of 500 mrem [5 mSv], because the intake of 1 ALI results in a CEDE of 5 rem [0.05 Sv]) and that minors and declared pregnant women are not likely to receive a CEDE >100 mrem (1mSvc) (i.e., 2% of an ALI), monitoring of occupational intakes in these individuals would not be required. Appendix B to Part 20 specifies ALIs (in units of μCi) of radionuclides for occupational exposure. The ALIs in this appendix are the annual intakes of a given radionuclide that would result in either: (1) a CEDE of 5 rem (0.05 Sv) (stochastic ALI), or (2) a CEDE of 50 rem (0.5 Sv) to an organ or tissue (nonstochastic ALI). However, these ALIs are based on generalized metabolic and biochemical properties and are not recommended for use by licensees utilizing unsealed sources for which a written directive is needed. When specific information on the physical and biochemical properties of the radionuclides taken into the body or the behavior of the material in an individual is known, the licensee may use that information to calculate the CEDE (§ 20.1204 (c)).

An estimate of the maximum likely internal dose (i.e., CEDE) to an individual exposed to a radioactivity source (in rem) from internal exposure can be calculated as:

$$\mathbf{CEDE = Q \times 10^{-6} \times DCF,} \qquad (16\text{-}1)$$

where Q = activity handled (mCi), 10^{-6} = assumed fractional intake, and DCF = dose conversion factor (rem/mCi).

A common rule of thumb or heuristic is to assume that no more than 1 millionth of the activity being handled will become an intake to an individual working with radioactive material. This rule was developed for cases of worker intakes during normal workplace operations, worker intakes from accidental exposures, and public intakes from accidental airborne releases from a licensed facility. (*Note:* NRC licensing guidance, as given in NUREG-1556, Volume 9, Appendix U, "Release of Patients Administered Radioactive Materials," recommended a value of 10^{-5} for the assumed fractional intake without justification, except to add a degree of conservatism to the calculation; see additional discussion in section 16.4.2.2.) The DCF converts intakes in millicuries to an internal CEDE, and values are available for both the ingestion and inhalation pathway in Environmental Protection Agency Federal Guidance Report No. 11, *Limiting Values of Radionuclide Intake and Air Concentration and Dose Conversion Factors for Inhalation, Submersion, and Ingestion* (Washington, DC: Environmental

Protection Agency; 1988). These values and the resulting CEDEs for the most commonly used radionuclides in radiopharmaceutical therapy are shown in Table 16.1.

It is important to note that, because of differences in biodistribution, the DCFs used to generate Table 16.1 are accurate for the radionuclide but not necessarily for the specific radiopharmaceutical intake. In addition, the fact that all commercially available preparations of Na ^{131}I (capsules and liquid) are now stabilized against volatility was not taken into account. Thus, the inhalation CEDE values are overly conservative. Nevertheless, all values of the CEDE, with the exception of those associated with the use of unstabilized ^{131}I, are extremely low and demonstrate that the dose component resulting from internal intake is not likely to pose any danger for individuals as a result of therapeutic radionuclide procedures. For example, the highest estimated CEDE (0.032 mrem) results from ingestion associated with the use of 30 mCi ^{90}Y (e.g., use of Food and Drug Administration–approved Zevalin [ibritumomab tiuxetan] for treatment of patients with non-Hodgkin's lymphoma). To exceed the 10%-of-the-ALI threshold (i.e., 500 mrem CEDE) that requires occupational intake monitoring, an adult worker would have to perform more than 62 of these procedures per day. A minor or declared pregnant woman would have to perform more than 12 procedures per day to exceed the 100-mrem CEDE threshold. Both scenarios are unlikely. It is essential to point out that intakes of ^{131}I in personnel have been monitored for years with very few significant occurrences. This is, no doubt, a result of the stabilization of the preparations against volatility.

Therefore, licensees are not required to routinely monitor the internal component of the occupational radiation dose and can demonstrate compliance with the annual dose limits by monitoring only external exposure. A licensee is, however, required to assess the need for ^{131}I intake monitoring, particularly when liquid dosages are manipulated, dosages are very large, or a licensee uses unstabilized ^{131}I in large amounts (e.g., for radiolabeling of antibodies). In such cases, an internal dose assessment may be necessary.

16.1.3 Suggested Procedures for Compliance

The model procedures given in Chapter 9 should be followed. The types and quantities of radioactive material properly manipulated for therapeutic radionuclide medical uses do not provide a reasonable possibility for internal intake by workers, with the possible exception of unstabilized ^{131}I used for radiolabeling antibodies and other agents. Workers using these radiopharmaceuticals should perform labeling procedures in a fume hood, and their thyroids should be monitored for radioactivity intake. This can be accomplished using standard counting techniques over the thyroid gland with a thyroid uptake probe. The bioassay procedure should provide for baseline, routine, emergency, and follow-up measures.

TABLE 16.1
DCFs and Resulting CEDEs for Commonly Used Radionuclides in Radiopharmaceutical Therapy

Radionuclide activity (mCi)	Ingestion		Inhalation	
	DCF (rem/mCi)	CEDE (mrem)	DCF (rem/mCi)	CEDE (mrem)
^{32}P (4)	0.88	0.0035	0.61	0.0024
^{89}Sr (4)	0.93	0.0037	0.65	0.0026
^{90}Y (30)	1.08	0.032	0.79	0.024
^{131}I (100)	53.28	5.3	32.89	3.3
^{153}Sm (70)	0.30	0.021	0.20	0.014

DCF = dose conversion factor; CEDE = committed effective dose equivalent.

16.2 Radiation Surveys

16.2.1 Pertinent Regulations

10 CFR 35.70 Surveys of ambient radiation exposure rate.

Licensees must survey with a radiation detection survey instrument at the end of each day of use all areas where unsealed byproduct material requiring a written directive was prepared for use or administered.

Licensees do not need to perform these surveys in areas where patients or human research subjects are confined when they cannot be released under § 35.75.

A record of each survey must be retained in accordance with § 35.2070.

16.2.2 Discussion of the Requirements

Licensees are required to perform daily surveys in all areas used for the preparation and administration of radiopharmaceuticals for which a written directive is required. When the licensee administers radio-pharmaceuticals requiring a written directive in a patient's room, the licensee is not required to perform a daily survey. Daily radiation surveys are also not required in areas where patients or human research subjects are confined when they cannot be released under § 35.75.

16.2.3 Suggested Procedures for Compliance

The model procedures given in Chapter 9 should be followed. In addition, daily surveys must be performed and records retained in all areas used during preparation and administration of radiopharmaceuticals for which a written directive is required. If radionuclide administration occurs in a patient's room, daily surveys are not required. Moreover, any areas in which patients or human research subjects are confined when they cannot be released under § 35.75 are not required to be surveyed. However, area surveys are required before releasing for unrestricted use the room of a patient who was confined in accordance with § 35.75 (see section 16.5). Patients treated as inpatients for medical and not radiation safety reasons (i.e., those patients who are releasable under § 35.75) generate no special requirements for radiation surveys. Also, rooms occupied by these patients need not be posted with caution signs pursuant to 10 CFR 20.1903(b). These patients are not considered to be sources of external exposures.

16.3 Written Directives

16.3.1 Pertinent Regulations

10 CFR 35.27 Supervision.

Licensees must instruct all supervised individuals in the licensee's written directive procedures and require that the supervised individuals follow these procedures.

10 CFR 35.40 Written directives.

A written directive must be dated and signed by an authorized user (AU) physician before the administration of Na ^{131}I in amounts >30 μCi (1.11 MBq) or any other therapeutic dosage of unsealed byproduct material.

If, because of the emergent nature of the patient's condition, a delay to provide a written directive would jeopardize his or her health, an oral directive is acceptable. The information contained in the oral directive must be documented as soon as possible in writing in the patient's record. A written directive must be prepared within 48 hours of the oral directive.

The written directive must contain the patient's or human research subject's name and the following information:

(1) The dosage for any administration of quantities >30 μCi (1.11 MBq) Na ^{131}I; or

(2) The radioactive drug, dosage, and route of administration for any administration of a therapeutic dosage of unsealed byproduct material other than Na ^{131}I.

A written revision to an existing written directive may be made if the revision is dated and signed by an AU before the administration of the dosage. If, because of the patient's condition, a delay to provide a written revision to an existing written directive would jeopardize his or her health, an oral revision is acceptable. The oral revision must be documented as soon as possible in the patient's record. A revised written directive must be signed by the AU within 48 hours of the oral revision. The licensee must retain a copy of the written directive in accordance with § 35.2040.

10 CFR 35.41 Procedures for administrations requiring a written directive.

For any administration requiring a written directive, the licensee must develop, implement, and maintain written procedures to provide high confidence that:

(1) The patient's or human research subject's identity is verified before each administration; and

(2) Each administration is in accordance with the written directive.

At a minimum, the required written procedures must verify:

(1) The identity of the individual; and

(2) That the administration is in accordance with the written directive.

The licensee must retain a copy of the required procedures in accordance with § 35.2041.

16.3.2 Discussion of the Requirements

Licensees must develop, maintain, and implement procedures for dosage administrations that require written directives. Licensees must instruct all supervised individuals in the licensee's written directive procedures and require that the supervised individuals follow these procedures. Written directives must be prepared for any administration of Na ^{131}I in amounts >30 μCi (1.11 MBq) and for a therapeutic dosage of any other radiopharmaceutical. The written directive must contain the information described in 10 CFR 35.40 and be retained in accordance with 10 CFR 35.2040. The AU physician may indicate a dosage range (instead of a single dosage) or a dosage that could deviate by plus or minus a specified percentage. Note that the NRC defines prescribed dosage in § 35.2, *Definitions*, as the specified activity or range of activity of unsealed byproduct material.

16.3.3 Suggested Procedures for Compliance

These procedures can be followed:

(1) Written directives must contain the patient's or human research subject's name and:

a. The dosage for any administration of quantities >30 μCi (1.11 MBq) Na ^{131}I; or

b. The radioactive drug, dosage, and route of administration for a therapeutic dosage other than Na ^{131}I.

It is recommended that the AU physician write the written directive in such a manner as to indicate a range of dosage or a dosage that is allowed to vary by plus or minus a specified percentage. A simple form should be developed with blanks for all the required information to simplify the written directive process.

(2) An AU must sign and date a written directive before the administration of any therapeutic dosage. A copy of the written directive must be retained. Written directives may also be maintained in patients' charts.

(3) Before administering a dosage, the patient's or human research subject's identity will be verified positively as the individual named in the written directive. This may be accomplished by examination of the patient's identification bracelet, hospital identification card, driver's license, or Social Security card or by asking the patient to state his or her name. It is best to avoid procedures in which the patient can answer "yes" or "no."

(4) The specific details of the administration will be verified, including the dosage, in accordance with the written directive. All components of the written directive (e.g., radionuclide, total dosage) will be confirmed to be in agreement with the written directive before dosage administration. This confirmation should include determination of the dosage and checking the labeled vial or syringe containing the therapeutic dosage.

(5) When deviations from the written directive or the established procedures are found, the cause of each deviation and the action required to prevent recurrence should be identified. *Note:* If the deviation constitutes a medical event, the licensee must report it to the NRC no later than the next calendar day (see § 35.3045 in section 16.7).

(6) All supervised individuals will be instructed in and required to follow the written directive procedures.

(7) The AU may wish to be present during a therapeutic administration. This is also helpful in that the AU can, when warranted, easily acknowledge and approve any necessary deviations from the written directive. (Oral revision to an existing written directive is only acceptable if a delay in order to provide a

written revision would jeopardize the patient's health.) AU presence and use of oral revision, when warranted, greatly reduces the possibility of medical events, because the dose is administered in accordance with the AU's directive regardless of the existing written directive. The AU can later modify the written directive to reflect the change.

(8) Conduct periodic reviews to ensure that written directive procedures are effective.

16.4 Release of Individuals Containing Unsealed Byproduct Material

16.4.1 Pertinent Regulations

10 CFR 35.75 Release of individuals containing unsealed byproduct material or implants containing byproduct material.

Licensees may authorize the release from their control of any individual who has been administered unsealed byproduct material if the TEDE to any other individual from exposure to the released individual is not likely to exceed 0.5 rem (5 mSv).

Licensees must provide the released individual or the individual's parent or guardian with instructions, including written instructions, on actions recommended to maintain doses to others as low as is reasonably achievable (ALARA) if the TEDE to any other individual is likely to exceed 0.1 rem (1 mSv).

If the TEDE to a nursing infant or child could exceed 0.1 rem (1 mSv) if breast feeding continues uninterrupted, the instructions must also include:

(1) Guidance on the interruption or discontinuation of breast feeding; and

(2) Information on the potential consequences, if any, of failure to follow the guidance.

Licensees must maintain a record of the basis for authorizing patient release in accordance with § 35.2075(a) and a record of instruction provided to a female who is breast feeding, in accordance with § 35.2075(b).

16.4.2 Discussion of the Requirements

NRC regulations (10 CFR 35.75) for the release of patients administered radioactive material authorize such release according to a dose-based limit (i.e., the dose to other individuals exposed to the patient). The dose-based limit, which replaces the previous activity- or dose-rate–based release limit (<30 mCi or <5 mrem/h at 1 meter), better expresses the NRC's primary concern for public health and safety. A licensee may now release a patient if the TEDE to another individual from exposure to that patient is not likely to exceed 0.5 rem (5 mSv). Compliance with this dose limit has been demonstrated by licensees by either using a default table for activity or dose rate provided in NUREG-1556, Volume 9 (which supercedes Regulatory Guide 8.39) or by performing a patient-specific dose calculation. A regulatory analysis on the new dose-based limit concludes that it is safe according to standard radiation protection principles, results in less hospitalization (thus significantly reducing national health care costs), and has personal and psychological benefits for patients and their families (Schneider S, McGuire SA. *Regulatory Analysis on Criteria for the Release of Patients Administered Radioactive Material.* NUREG-1492 [Final Report]. Washington, DC: U. S. Nuclear Regulatory Commission; 1996).

In addition to demonstrating compliance with the 0.5 rem (5 mSv) TEDE limit, the licensee must:

(1) Provide written instructions to the released patient or the patient's parent or guardian on actions recommended to maintain ALARA doses to other individuals if the TEDE to any other individual is likely to exceed 0.1 rem (1 mSv). If the dose to a breast feeding infant or child could exceed 0.1 rem (1 mSv), these instructions must also include guidance on interruption or discontinuation of breast feeding and information on the potential consequences, if any, of failure to follow this guidance.

(2) Maintain records according to § 35.2075(a) for 3 years after the date of patient release, documenting the basis for patient release, if the TEDE is calculated by:

a. Using retained activity rather than the activity administered;

b. Using an occupancy factor <0.25 at 1 meter;

c. Using the biological or effective half-life; or

d. Considering the shielding by tissue (i.e., using measured dose rate).

(3) Maintain records according to § 35.2075(b), for 3 years after the date of patient release, documenting that instruction was provided to breast feeding women if radiation dose to infant or child from continued breast feeding could result in a TEDE >0.5 rem (5 mSv).

16.4.2.1 External Dose Component

The following equation can be used to estimate the dose an individual is likely to receive from exposure to a released patient:

$$D(\infty) = \frac{(34.6 \times \Gamma \times Q_0 \times T_p \times E)}{r^2}, \quad (16\text{-}1)$$

where $D(\infty)$ = total dose in millirems from exposure to gamma radiation; Γ = exposure rate constant (mR cm^2/mCi h); Q_0 = administered activity in mCi; T_p = physical half-life of radionuclide in days; E = occupancy factor at 1 meter = 0.25; and r = distance from patient = 1 meter = 100 cm.

This "patient release" equation, which is based on the physical half-life of the radionuclide (i.e., no biological elimination is assumed), is essentially the same as that introduced in 1970 in the National Council on Radiation Protection and Measurements (NCRP) Report No. 37, *Precautions in the Management of Patients Who Have Received Therapeutic Amounts of Radionuclides* (Bethesda, MD: NCRP; 1970), with the exception of the occupancy factor. The selection of an occupancy factor of 0.25 at 1 meter is based on professional judgment about time–distance combinations that are believed likely to occur when appropriate instructions are given to minimize time spent close to the patient.

Using the various half-lives and exposure rate constants for the radionuclides commonly employed in radionuclide therapy, equation 16-1 (upon rearrangement and substitution of 500 mrem for $D(\infty)$, 100 cm for r, and 0.25 for E) can be used to determine the maximum allowable administered activities and/or dose rates at 1 meter for authorizing patient release based on the 0.5 rem (5 mSv) TEDE limit pursuant to § 35.75(a).

16.4.2.1.1 Release Based on Administered Activity:

$$Q_0(\text{mCi}) < D(\infty) \times \frac{r^2}{34.6 \times \Gamma \times T_p \times E} < \frac{5.78 \times 10^5}{\Gamma \times T_p} \quad (16\text{-}2)$$

16.4.2.1.2 Release Based on Measured Dose Rate at 1 Meter:

Because dose rate at 1 meter (DR) $= \frac{(\Gamma \times Q_0)}{r^2}$,

$$\text{DR (mrem/h)} < \frac{D(\infty)}{34.6 \times T_p \times E} < 57.8/T_p \quad (16\text{-}3)$$

The appropriate parameters and release activities and dose rates for the most commonly used radionuclides in radiopharmaceutical therapy are given in Table 16.2.

In compliance with the dose limit in 10 CFR 35.75(a), licensees may release patients from their control if the activity administered or measured dose rate at 1 meter is no greater than the values listed in Table 16.2. If release is based on administered activity,

TABLE 16.2
Maximum Activities and Dose Rates for Authorizing Patient Release

Radionuclide	Half-life (days)	Γ (mR cm^2/mCi h)	Activity (mCi)	Dose rate (mrem/h)
^{32}P	14.29	4.05*	9988	4.0
^{89}Sr	50.5	3.14*	3645	1.1
^{90}Y	2.67	5.64*	38,385	21.6
^{131}I	8.04	2200	33	7.2
^{153}Sm	1.946	425	699	29.7

* NRC licensing guidance, given in NUREG-1556, Volume 9, does not determine activity and dose rate limits for beta emitters "because of the minimal exposures to members of the public resulting from activities normally administered for diagnostic or therapeutic purposes." The exposure rate constants given in this table for the pure beta-emitting radionuclides ^{32}P, ^{89}Sr, and ^{90}Y are specific bremsstrahlung constants (Zanzonico PB, Binkert BL, Goldsmith SJ. Bremsstrahlung radiation exposure from pure ß-ray emitters. *J Nucl Med.* 1999; 40:1024–1028).

no record is required. If release is based on measured dose rate, a record is required, because the release is based on considering shielding by tissue. Patient instructions are only required if the TEDE to individuals is likely to exceed 0.1 rem (1 mSv). This would correspond to 1/5 of the values in Table 16.2, because these values were determined based on a TEDE of 0.5 rem (5 mSv). For example, it is easily determined that the activity values to ensure that individuals exposed to the patient are not likely to receive a dose >0.1 rem (1 mSv) from ^{32}P, ^{89}Sr, ^{90}Y, ^{131}I, and ^{153}Sm are 1,998 mCi (73.9 GBq), 729 mCi (27.0 GBq), 7,677 mCi (284.0 GBq), 7 mCi (0.26 GBq), and 140 mCi (5.18 GBq), respectively. Because patients will be administered activities less than these values, with the exception of patients receiving ^{131}I, all patients receiving pure beta-emitting radionuclides or ^{153}Sm for radionuclide therapy are releasable. No records or instructions are required.

The release approach taken so far has utilized the physical half-life but not the effective half-life of the radionuclide. This is reasonable for the beta-emitting radionuclides and ^{153}Sm but is inappropriate for Na ^{131}I. Therapy patients receiving ^{131}I do not retain radioactivity for the physical half-life of the radionuclide; instead, the administered activity is rapidly excreted.

As a result, patient-specific dose calculations should be performed for ^{131}I therapy patients to provide a more complete and appropriate estimation of dose to individuals likely to be exposed to the patient. These calculations may involve the use of any of the following four patient-specific factors:

(1) Retained activity;

(2) Occupancy or exposure factor (E) <0.25 at 1 meter;

(3) T_{eff} or T_b (i.e., measured biological elimination); or

(4) Attenuation/shielding by tissue (i.e., measured dose rate).

It should be noted that the NRC has stated that in those instances for which a case-specific calculation applies to more than one patient release (that is, the calculation is case-specific for a class of patients), the calculation need not be performed again. In such a case, the record for a particular patient's release may reference the calculation for the class of patients.

16.4.2.1.3 Release of Patients Administered Na ^{131}I for Treatment of Thyroid Cancer and Hyperthyroidism

Equation 16-1 was modified in NUREG-1556, Volume 9, Appendix U, "Model Procedure for Release of Patients or Human Research Subjects Administered Radioactive Materials," in Supplement B, to account for the uptake and retention of the radionuclide by the patient in both the thyroid and the remainder of the body (i.e., thyroidal and extrathyroidal terms). The modification also included a term to account for the fact that during the initial hours after administration of the radiolabeled material, the patient may not void and the activity therefore is not removed from the body. The following equation was used:

$$D(\infty) = [34.6 \times \Gamma \times Q_0] / (100\ \text{cm})^2 \{E_1 T_p (0.8) (1 - e^{-0.693(T_{NV})/T_p}) + e^{-0.693(T_{NV})/T_p} E_2 F_1 T_{1eff} + e^{-0.693(T_{NV})/T_p} E_2 F_2 T_{2eff}\}, \quad (16\text{-}4)$$

where E_1 = occupancy factor for nonvoid period = 0.75; T_{NV} = nonvoid period in days = 0.33 (8 hours); E_2 = occupancy factor from 8 hours to total decay = 0.25; F_1 = extrathyroidal uptake fraction = 0.20 in hyperthyroid patients = 0.95 in thyroid cancer patients (post-thyroidectomy); T_{1eff} = effective half-life of extrathyroidal component = 0.32 days in hyperthyroid patients = 0.32 days in thyroid cancer patients (post-thyroidectomy); F_2 = thyroidal uptake fraction = 0.80 in hyperthyroid patients = 0.05 in thyroid cancer patients (post-thyroidectomy); and T_{2eff} = effective half-life of thyroidal component = 5.2 days in hyperthyroid patients = 7.3 days in thyroid cancer patients (post-thyroidectomy).

Note: According to the NRC, these effective half-life and uptake fraction parameter values are "acceptable" values to be used in "class-specific" dose calculations for patients with thyroid cancer and hyperthyroidism. Thus, individual dose calculations need not be performed on a case-by-case basis for these patients, unless a specific patient's situation warrants the use of parameter values different from those used in equation 16-4.

Equation 16-4 can be solved for the maximum allowable administered activities and dose rates at 1 meter for authorizing patient release based on the 0.5 rem (5 mSv) TEDE limit. These values are given in Table 16.3 for occupancy factors (E_2) of 0.25 and 0.125.

TABLE 16.3

Maximum Activities and Dose Rates at 1 Meter for Authorizing Release of Patients Treated for Thyroid Cancer and Hyperthyroidism*

Releasable activity (mCi) E_2 =	0.25	0.125	Releasable dose rate (mrem/h) E_2 =	0.25	0.125
Thyroid cancer	221	303	Thyroid cancer	48.5	66.7
Hyperthyroidism	57	101	Hyperthyroidism	12.4	22.3

*Based on NUREG-1556, Volume 9.
E_2 = occupancy factor from 8 h to total decay; an occupancy factor of 0.125 must be justified (e.g., patient lives alone and expects no visitors).

Licensees may choose to use the values in Table 16.3 as their basis for patient release. These values for activity and dose rate at 1 meter can be applied to all patients, unless a specific patient situation does not match the assumption made for the "class of patients" calculation.

This approach is highly conservative and may be unnecessarily restrictive. It must be noted that several assumptions were made in assigning values to the parameters used in equation 16-4 in determining patient release activities and dose rates. These include:

(1) Use of the exposure rate constant and the inverse square law, a point-source based model, which does not account for attenuation or distribution of the radiation in the body of the patient;
(2) Use of an 8-hour nonvoid period;
(3) Use of an occupancy factor of 0.75 during nonvoid period; and
(4) Use of representative values for uptake fractions and effective half-lives for thyroidal and extrathyroidal components.

In addition, dosimeter measurements obtained in 65 household members of 30 patients who received outpatient ^{131}I therapy for thyroid carcinoma indicated that the measured radiation dose was on average a factor of 10 lower than the radiation dose predicted based on equation 16-4 (Grigsby PW, Siegel BA, Baker S, Eichling JO. Radiation exposure from outpatient radioactive iodine [^{131}I] therapy for thyroid carcinoma. *JAMA.* 2000;283:2272–2274).

Licensees may therefore choose to perform more realistic calculations and not use Table 16.3. Dose rates should be measured, and allowable release limits should not be based on the use of an exposure rate constant that does not account for radionuclide distribution and patient attenuation. To account for distribution and attenuation of ^{131}I in the patient, for example, a value of 1,700 mR cm^2/mCi h could be used in place of the value of 2,200 given in Table 16.2 (Carey JE, Kumpuris TM, Wrobel MC. Release of patients containing therapeutic dosages of iodine-131 from hospitals. *J Nucl Med Technol.* 1995;23:144–149). Smaller values for the nonvoid period (0–1 hour for well-hydrated patients) are justified and could be used. Similarly, an occupancy factor (E_1) of 0.25 could be used for the nonvoid period, if any. Finally, licensees may choose to determine the biokinetics in an individual patient to use measured values for the uptake fractions and effective half-times. Use of any of these more patient-specific approaches will permit less conservative release limits, if so desired.

For example, using equation 16-4 and substituting an exposure rate constant equal to 1,700 mR cm^2/mCi h, a nonvoid period of 1 hour, and an occupancy factor of 0.25 during this period, the maximum allowable activities and dose rates for authorizing patient release are given in Table 16.4.

Licensees may choose to use the values in Table 16.4 as their basis for patient release. The maximum activity and dose rate values are higher in Table 16.4 than in Table 16.3 because of the use of less conservative and more realistic parameter values in equation 16-4.

The usual instructions given to patients released under the old regulations should be given to these higher activity releasable patients. However, these instructions should be in place for a longer period of

TABLE 16.4

Alternative Maximum Activities and Dose Rates at 1 Meter for Authorizing Release of Patients Treated for Thyroid Cancer and Hyperthyroidism*

Conditions	**Releasable activity (mCi)**		**Condition**	**Releasable dose rate (mrem/h)**	
E_2 =	**0.25**	**0.125**	**E_2 =**	**0. 25**	**0.125**
Thyroid cancer	493	954	Thyroid cancer	83.8	162.2
Hyperthyroidism	80	160	Hyperthyroidism	13.7	27.2

*Based on methodology described in this chapter.

E_2 = occupancy factor from 8 h to total decay; an occupancy factor of 0.125 must be justified (e.g., patient lives alone and expects no visitors).

time. In 1987, the Society of Nuclear Medicine, in collaboration with the NRC, published a pamphlet, *Guidelines for Patients Receiving Radioiodine Treatment,* that provided information for patients receiving treatment with radioiodine. The NRC still considers the instructions in this pamphlet to be acceptable, provided the times given for the instructions are appropriate for the activity and medical condition.

However, today radioactive articles in the household trash of patients are appearing at solid waste landfills that have installed radiation monitors to prevent the entry of any detectable radioactivity. Alarms are going off around the country. These monitors are set to alarm at extremely low activity levels (Siegel JA, Sparks RB. Radioactivity appearing at landfills in household trash of nuclear medicine patients: Much ado about nothing? *Health Phys.* 2002;82:367–372).

Although the NRC has stated that the low activity levels potentially contained in any radioactive household waste of patients released in accordance with § 35.75 pose an insignificant hazard to the public health and safety or to the environment, professionals can take steps to avoid issues with landfill owners and operators and even individual states. It is probably wise to instruct patients to avoid or minimize use of items that cannot be disposed of via plumbing (toilet, sink, dishwasher, washing machine), such as plastic utensils and paper plates.

16.4.2.1.4 Release of Patients Administred Gamma-Emitting Radionuclides for Treatment of Cancers Other than Thyroid

The prime example in this category is the release of patients receiving radioimmunotherapy with ^{131}I-labeled monoclonal antibodies. A tracer dosage is usually administered to determine total body effective half-time, which is highly patient dependent. This half-time value is used to determine the appropriate therapeutic dosage. After the therapeutic administration, a dose rate measurement at 1 m should be obtained. Licensees may then calculate the maximum likely dose to exposed individuals on a case-by-case basis using the 2 patient-specific parameters of total body effective half-time and dose rate at 1 m.

Many references are available to help guide the practitioner in the performance of a patient-specific dose calculation for patients receiving ^{131}I-labeled monoclonal antibodies, as well as Na ^{131}I, and in the issuance of release instructions to such radionuclide therapy patients. These include:

(1) Siegel JA. Outpatient radionuclide therapy. In: *Radiation Protection in Medicine: Contemporary Issues.* Proceedings of the Thirty-Fifth Annual Meeting of the National Council on Radiation Protection and Measurements. Proceedings No. 21. Bethesda, MD: National Council on Radiation Protection and Measurements; 1999:187–199.

(2) Zanzonico PB, Siegel JA, St. Germain J. A generalized algorithm for determining the time of release and the duration of post-release radiation precautions following radionuclide therapy. *Health Phys.* 2000;78:648–659.

(3) Siegel JA, Kroll S, Regan D, Kaminski MS, Wahl RL. A practical methodology for patient release after tositumomab and ^{131}I tositumomab therapy. *J Nucl Med.* 2002;43:354–363.

(4) Siegel JA, Marcus CS, Sparks RB. Calculating the absorbed dose to others from the radioactive

patient: line source model versus point source model. *J Nucl Med.* 2002;43:1241–1244.

(5) Marcus CS. Considerations in determining whether or not patients may be given significant quantities of radiopharmaceuticals as outpatients. Accessed through the California chapter of the American College of Nuclear Physicians Web site at www.acnp-cal.org/ radiopharmaceuticals.html.

16.4.2.2 Internal Dose Component

So far in this discussion, the TEDE has been assumed to be exclusively from the external radiation dose. The internal radiation dose component, referred to as the CEDE, has not been considered. It must be pointed out that the NRC does not require determination of the internal dose contribution if it is likely to be <10% of the external dose.

A common rule of thumb is to assume that no more than 1 millionth of the activity being handled will become an intake to an individual working with the material. This rule of thumb, or heuristic, was developed for cases of worker intakes during normal workplace operations, worker intakes from accidental exposures, and public intakes from accidental airborne releases from a facility (Brodsky A. Resuspension factors and probabilities of intake of material in process [or is 10^{-6} a magic number in health physics?]. *Health Phys.* 1980;39:992–1000), but it does not specifically apply for cases of intake by an individual exposed to a patient. Limited data are available for thyroid uptakes in family members exposed to Na ^{131}I patients. Two studies (Buchan RCT, Brindle JM. Radioiodine therapy to outpatients—the contamination hazard. *Br J Radiol.* 1970:43:479–482; and Jacobson AP, Plato PA, Toeroek D. Contamination of the home environment by patients treated with iodine-131: initial results. *Am J Public Health.* 1978;68:230–235) on the intakes of individuals exposed to patients administered ^{131}I indicated that intakes were generally on the order of 1 millionth of the activity administered to the patient and that internal doses were far below external doses. The *maximum* observed fractional internal intakes for these two studies were 0.2×10^{-5} and 0.4×10^{-5}, respectively.

An estimate of the maximum likely CEDE from internal exposure can be calculated according to:

$$\mathbf{CEDE = Q \times 10^{-6} \times DCF,} \tag{16-5}$$

where CEDE = maximum likely internal CEDE to the individual exposed to the patient, in rem; Q = activity administered to the patient, in millicuries; 10^{-6} = assumed fractional intake; DCF = dose conversion factor to convert an intake in millicuries to an internal CEDE = 53 rem/mCi for Na^{131}I (Eckerman KF, Wolbarst AB, Richardson ACB. *Limiting Values of Radionuclide Intake and Air Concentration and Dose Conversion Factors for Inhalation, Submersion, and Ingestion.* Federal Guidance Report No. 11. Washington, DC: U.S. Environmental Protection Agency; 1988).

Note: NRC licensing guidance (i.e., NUREG-1556, Vol. 9, Appendix U) recommended a value of 10^{-5} for the assumed fractional intake to account for the most highly exposed individual and to add a degree of conservatism to the calculation. However, no such "highly exposed" individual has been found, and no documentation substantiates that this conservative approach is advisable, necessary, or accurate.

Example: Using the ingestion pathway, calculate the maximum internal dose to a person exposed to a patient who has been administered 200 mCi Na ^{131}I. Substituting the appropriate values into equation 16-5, the maximum internal dose to the exposed individual is:

$$\mathbf{CEDE = 200\ mCi \times 10^{-6} \times 53\ rem/mCi = 10.6\ mrem.} \tag{16-6}$$

In this case, the internal dose is 10.6 mrem. Therefore, the external dose to any exposed individual must not be >489.4 mrem (500 – 10.6 mrem). To be <10% of the external gamma dose and to maintain the TEDE to <500 mrem, the CEDE must be <45 mrem (even if the maximum observed fractional intake of 4×10^{-6} was used in the calculation, the resulting CEDE of 42.4 mrem is within the 45 mrem limit). Because the internal dose is likely to be <10% of the external gamma dose, it need not be taken into account in the calculations for patient release.

The NCRP addressed the risk of intake of radionuclides from patients' secretions and excreta in NCRP Commentary No. 11, *Dose Limits for Individuals who Receive Exposure from Radionuclide Therapy Patients,* and concluded: "Thus, a contamination incident that could lead to a significant intake of radioactive material is very unlikely."

16.4.3 Suggested Procedures for Compliance

Licensees can authorize patient release after radionuclide therapy using the activity and/or dose rate limits given in Table 16.2 for beta-emitting radionuclides and ^{153}Sm. The values of activity and dose rate in Tables 16.3 and 16.4 can be used as guidance for many patients (i.e., the case-specific calculations performed to generate these tables may apply to more than one patient release). Either a specific calculation should be made by the AU or by a qualified individual, or this individual should verify that the patient's situation matches the assumptions made for a previous calculation for a class of patients. The record for a specific patient's release could reference the calculation performed for the class of patients. Records must be kept if the basis for authorizing patient release involves Tables 16.3 and 16.4. Records are not required for patients receiving beta-emitting radionuclides or ^{153}Sm-ethylenediamine tetramethylenephosphonic acid (EDTMP).

Note: Make sure that the appropriate occupancy factor is being used; generally this value can be set at 0.25. If an occupancy factor <0.25 is used (e.g., 0.125), it must be justified and recorded. Licensees may use occupancy factors >0.25 (e.g., 0.5) if appropriate for a particular patient's release, without the need for recordkeeping. Licensees may also choose to measure individual patient biokinetics and use more detailed analyses of distances and exposure times relevant to individuals likely to be in the vicinity of the patient.

Any patients not releasable in accordance with § 35.75 must be hospitalized (see Section 16.5).

For Na ^{131}I and other ^{131}I-labeled radiopharmaceuticals, the practitioner may also use the references cited in Section 16.4.2.1 as a guide in implementing release limits that are even more patient-specific, if so desired. The internal dose component does not have to be taken into account. The TEDE is almost entirely the result of the external dose component.

Patient instructions, if required (no regulations require instructions for patients receiving beta-emitters or ^{153}Sm), may include:

(1) Maintaining distance from other individuals;
(2) Separate sleeping arrangements;
(3) Minimizing time in public places;
(4) Precautions to reduce spread of radioactive contamination (control of body fluid contami nation is an important concern for Na ^{131}I; it is much less problematic for ^{131}I-labeled antibod ies, beta-emitting radionuclides, and ^{153}Sm-EDTMP;
(5) Precautions to reduce likelihood of radioactive household trash appearing at solid waste landfills (at least until the landfill issue is resolved); and
(6) Length of time each of the instructions should be in effect.

The AU physician must be professionally satisfied that patient compliance with any instructions is highly likely before authorizing patient release.

It is generally best to stop lactation in any patient given Na ^{131}I. Stopping lactation for 3 weeks is sufficient to ensure cessation of milk production and no extra radiation absorbed dose to the breasts after treatment. In the event that a radiation dose to an infant needs to be calculated because of radioactive breast milk ingestion, we recommend using data from the publication by Stabin and Breitz (Breast milk excretion of radiopharmaceuticals: mechanisms, findings, and radiation dosimetry. *J Nucl Med.* 2000;41:862–873).

Patients who are breast feeding should not receive radionuclide therapy. If the patient is breast feeding, additional instructions should include appropriate recommendations on whether to interrupt breast feeding and the length of time to interrupt breast feeding, or, if necessary, the discontinuation of breast feeding. The instructions should include information on the consequences, if any, of failure to follow the breast feeding guidance. Licensees should note that the required instructions are not in any way intended to interfere with the discretion and judgment of the physician in specifying detailed instructions and recommendations.

16.5 Safety Procedures for Treatment When Patients Are Hospitalized

16.5.1 Pertinent Regulations

10 CFR 20.1301 Dose limits for individual members of the public.

The TEDE to individual members of the public must not exceed 0.1 rem (1 mSv) in a year, and the dose in any unrestricted area from external sources must not exceed 2 mrem (0.02 mSv) in any 1 hour.

Note: The yearly dose limit does not include exposure from radionuclide therapy patients who are released in accordance with § 35.75, and these patients are not regarded as "external sources."

A licensee may permit visitors to an individual who cannot be released under § 35.75 to receive a radiation dose >0.1 rem (1 mSv) if:

(1) The radiation dose received does not exceed 0.5 rem (5 mSv); and
(2) The AU has determined before the visit that it is appropriate.

10 CFR 20.1302 Compliance with dose limits for individual members of the public.

A licensee must make or cause to be made, as appropriate, surveys of radiation levels in unrestricted and controlled areas to demonstrate compliance with the dose limits for individual members of the public in § 20.1301.

10 CFR 20.1501 General.

A licensee must make or cause to be made surveys that:

(1) May be necessary to comply with applicable Part 20 regulations; and
(2) Are reasonable under the circumstances to evaluate the magnitude and extent of radiation levels, concentrations or quantities of radioactive material, and potential radiological hazards.

10 CFR 35.315 Safety precautions.

For each patient or human research subject who cannot be released under § 35.75, licensees must:

(1) Quarter the patient or human research subject in either:
    a. A private room with a private sanitary facility; or
    b. A room with a private sanitary facility, with another individual who also has received therapy with unsealed byproduct material and who also cannot be released under § 35.75.
(2) Visibly post the individual's room with a "Radioactive Materials" sign.
(3) Note on the door or in the individual's chart where and for how long visitors may stay in the room; and
(4) Either monitor material and items removed from the room to determine that their radioactivity cannot be distinguished from natural background levels with a radiation detection survey instrument set on its most sensitive scale and with no interposed shielding *or* handle the material and items as radioactive waste.

Licensees must notify the radiation safety officer (RSO) or designee and the AU as soon as possible when a patient or human research subject has a medical emergency or dies.

16.5.2 Discussion of the Requirements

Certain radionuclide therapy patients may have to be hospitalized for a variety of reasons (e.g., they are unable to care for themselves or unlikely to follow instructions). Licensees must develop and implement procedures to ensure that in the event that a radionuclide therapy patient cannot be released in accordance with § 35.75, access to treatment rooms can be restricted and exposure rates from confined patients will be limited to maintain doses to occupational workers and members of the public within regulatory limits.

Licensees are required under 10 CFR 20.1501 to perform adequate surveys to evaluate the magnitude and extent of radiation levels. Therefore, licensees must evaluate exposure rates around patients who are hospitalized after the dosage administration (e.g., measured exposure rates, combination of measured and calculated exposure rates). To control exposures to individuals in accordance with 10 CFR Part 20, the licensee also should consider briefing patients on radiation safety procedures, limiting room access and visitor control, notification of medical staff in the event of problems, and other actions as applicable and consistent with good medical care. Safety instruction must be given to personnel caring for patients or human research subjects who cannot be released under § 35.75 (see section 16.8).

Regulatory requirements, the ALARA principle, good medical care, and access control should be considered when determining the location of the therapy patient's room. A corner room, for example, will keep dose rate concerns to a minimum in surrounding areas. It may be desirable for the designated therapy rooms to be on the same floor to minimize potential problems and assist in training efforts.

A licensee cannot legally force a patient who is required to be hospitalized after therapy to remain in the hospital. There is no requirement to contact the NRC if the patient leaves against medical advice.

16.5.3 Suggested Procedures for Compliance

For patients who cannot be released under 10 CFR 35.75, licensees must take the following steps:

(1) Provide a room with a private sanitary facility for patients treated with a radiopharmaceutical therapy dosage (*Note:* the room may be shared with another radiopharmaceutical therapy patient);

(2) Visibly post a "Radioactive Materials" sign on the patient's room, and note on the door or in the patient's chart where and for low long visitors may stay in the patient's room;

(3) Either monitor material and items removed from the patient's room (e.g., linens, surgical dressings) with a radiation detection survey instrument set on its most sensitive scale with no interposed shielding to determine that their radioactivity cannot be distinguished from the natural background radiation level *or* handle them as radioactive waste; and

(4) Notify the RSO or his or her designee and the AU as soon as possible when a patient has a medical emergency or dies.

A licensee may permit visitors to an individual who cannot be released under § 35.75 to receive a radiation dose >0.1 rem (1 mSv) if:

(1) The radiation dose received does not exceed 0.5 rem (5 mSv); and

(2) The authorized user has determined before the visit that it is appropriate.

Licensees are required to perform adequate surveys to evaluate the magnitude and extent of radiation levels. Therefore, licensees should evaluate the exposure rates around patients who are hospitalized, either by measured exposure rates or by a combination of measured and calculated exposure rates. The therapy rooms could also be "pre-evaluated" by placing a typical dosage at various locations in the room (e.g., on the empty bed, in the bathroom) and measuring the surrounding area dose rates, thereby alleviating the need to perform surveys for each patient.

Licensees also must perform surveys before the release of the room for unrestricted use. Licensees should be cognizant of the requirement to perform surveys to demonstrate that public dose limits are not exceeded. The TEDE to an individual member of the public must not exceed 0.1 rem (1 mSv) in a year, and the dose in any unrestricted area from external sources must not exceed 2 mrem (0.02 mSv) in any 1 hour. The surveys required before releasing the hospital room of a confined radionuclide therapy patient for use by other patients must demonstrate compliance with these public dose limits. No requirements in the revised Part 35 or elsewhere describe the level of removable contamination that could serve as an action level for wipe surveys. A value of 22,000 dpm/100 cm^2, suggested earlier in this volume, may bc used as a trigger level. To minimize potential contamination and facilitate cleanup if required based on radiation surveys, licensees may wish to cover appropriate areas of the room with absorbent paper or other suitable covering before patient dosage administration.

Licensees should know what steps to take if a therapy patient undergoes emergency surgery or dies. In such an event, it is necessary to ensure the safety of others attending the patient. As long as the patient's body remains unopened, the exposure received by anyone in close proximity is almost entirely from gamma radiation. The simple principles of time, distance, and shielding can be used to minimize potential exposures. When an operation or autopsy is to be performed, radiation dose to the hands and face is also possible from beta emissions, and avoidance of radiation contamination should be considered. Double thicknesses of surgical gloves or heavy rubber autopsy gloves may be used to reduce hand exposure from beta emissions. Procedures for emergency surgery or death can be found in Chapter 5 of NCRP Report No. 37, *Precautions in the Management of Patients Who Have Received Therapeutic Amounts of Radionuclides* (Bethesda, MD: NCRP; 1972).

16.6 Records

16.6.1 Pertinent Regulations

10 CFR 35.2040 Records of written directives.

Licensees must retain a copy of each written directive for 3 years.

10 CFR 35.2041 Records for procedures for administrations requiring a written directive.

Licensees must retain a copy of their procedures for administrations requiring a written directive for the duration of the license.

10 CFR 35.2070 Records of surveys for ambient radiation exposure rate.

Records of each survey required by § 35.70 must be retained for 3 years. The records must include the date of the survey, the results of the survey, the instrument used to make the survey, and the name of the individual who performed the survey.

10 CFR 35.2075 Records of the release of individuals containing unsealed byproduct material or implants containing byproduct material.

Records of the basis for authorizing the release of an individual must be retained if the TEDE is calculated by:

(1) Using the retained activity rather than the activity administered;

(2) Using an occupancy factor <0.25 at 1 meter;

(3) Using the biological or effective half-life; or

(4) Considering the shielding by tissue.

Records must also be retained, if applicable, indicating that instructions were provided to a woman who is breast feeding if the radiation dose to the infant or child from continued nursing could result in a TEDE >0.5 rem (5 mSv). All records must be retained for 3 years after the date of release of the individual.

10 CFR 35.2310 Records of safety instruction.

Records of safety instructions required by § 35.310 must be maintained for 3 years and must include, for each instruction session, a list of the topics covered, the date of the instruction, the name(s) of the attendee(s), and the name(s) of the individuals(s) who provided the instruction.

16.6.2 Discussion of the Requirements

The required records are self-explanatory.

16.6.3 Suggested Procedures for Compliance

Licensees should be able easily to develop forms for each of the required records based on the information in this chapter. Each required record must be legible throughout the specified retention period. The licensee must maintain adequate safeguards against tampering with and loss of these records.

16.7 Reports

16.7.1 Pertinent Regulations

Reports required pursuant to 10 CFR Parts 35.3045 and 35.3047 were discussed previously in this volume for diagnostic nuclear medicine but are reproduced here for emphasis.

10 CFR 20.2201 Reports of theft or loss of licensed material.

Licensees must notify the NRC Operation Center by telephone (301-951-0550):

(1) Immediately after the occurrence of any lost, stolen, or missing licensed material becomes known in a quantity ≥1,000 times that specified in Appendix C to Part 20 under such circumstances that it appears to the licensee that an exposure could result to persons in unrestricted areas; or

(2) Within 30 days after the occurrence of any lost, stolen, or missing licensed material becomes known in a quantity >10 times that specified in Appendix C to Part 20 (and is still missing at that time).

Quantities for the most commonly used radionuclides used in radiopharmaceutical therapy are given in Table 16.5.

TABLE 16.5

Quantities of Most Common Therapy Radionuclides to be Reported to the Nuclear Regulatory Commission if Lost or Stolen

Radionuclide	Quantity (mCi)*	
	Immediate	30 days
^{32}P	10	0.1
^{89}Sr	10	0.1
^{90}Y	10	0.1
^{131}I	1	0.01
^{153}Sm	100	1

*Quantities in the "Immediate" column require immediate NRC notification; quantities in the "30 days" column require NRC notification within 30 days.

Within 30 days after the telephone report, a written report must be made to the administrator of the appropriate NRC Regional Office, containing the following information: description of the licensed material involved, description of the circumstances under which the loss or theft occurred, statement of disposition or probable disposition of licensed material involved, exposures of individuals to radiations and circumstances under which the exposures occurred, actions that have been taken to recover the material, and procedures that have been adopted to ensure against a recurrence of the loss or theft. Names of individuals who may have received exposure to radiation must be stated in a separate and detachable part of the report.

10 CFR 35.3045 Report and notification of a medical event.

A licensee must report any event, except for an event resulting from patient intervention, in which the administration of licensed material results in:

(1) A dose that differs from the dose that would have resulted from the prescribed dosage by >5 rem EDE, 50 rem (0.05 Sv) to an organ or tissue, or 50 rem (0.5 Sv) shallow dose equivalent to the skin, and the total dosage delivered differs from prescribed dosage by 20% or more or falls outside prescribed dosage range; or

(2) A dose >5 rem (0.05 Sv) EDE, 50 rem to an organ or tissue, or 50 rem (0.5 Sv) shallow dose equivalent to the skin from any of the following: administration of wrong radioactive drug, administration of radioactive drug by wrong route of administration, administration of dosage to wrong individual or human research subject, or a leaking sealed source.

A licensee must report any event resulting from intervention of a patient or human research subject in which the administration of licensed material will result in unintended permanent functional damage to an organ or a physiological system, as determined by a physician. (Patient intervention means actions by the patient or human research subject, whether intentional or unintentional, such as dislodging or removing treatment devices or prematurely terminating the administration.)

A licensee must notify the NRC Operations Center by telephone no later than the next calendar day after discovery of the medical event. A written report must be submitted to the appropriate NRC Regional Office within 15 days and must include: licensee's name; name of prescribing physician; brief description of event; why event occurred; effect, if any, on individual(s) who received the administration; actions taken, if any, to prevent recurrence; and certification that licensee notified the individual (or responsible relative or guardian), and if not, why not. The report may not contain any information that could lead to identification of the individual. The licensee must also provide an annotated copy of the report to the referring physician no later than 15 days after the discovery of the event, with the name of the affected individual and his or her Social Security or other identification number.

A licensee must provide notification of the event to the referring physician and also notify the involved individual no later than 24 hours after discovery of the event, unless the referring physician personally informs the licensee either that he or she will inform the individual or that, based on medical judgment, telling the individual would be harmful. The licensee is not required to notify the individual without first consulting the referring physician. If the referring physician or affected individual cannot be reached within 24 hours, the licensee must notify the individual as soon as possible thereafter (if necessary, notification may be made to a responsible relative or guardian). The licensee may not delay any appropriate medical care for the individual. If a verbal notification is made, the licensee must inform the individual that a written description of the event can be obtained upon request.

Aside from notification, nothing in this requirement affects any rights or duties of licensees and physicians in relation to each other, to individuals affected by the medical event, or to those individuals' responsible relatives or guardians.

10 CFR 35.3047 Report and notification of a dose to an embryo/fetus or a nursing child.

A licensee must report any dose to an embryo/fetus that is >5 rem (0.05 Sv) dose equivalent resulting from the administration of byproduct material to a pregnant individual, unless the dose was specifically approved, in advance, by the authorized user.

A licensee must report any dose to a nursing child that is a result of an administration of byproduct material to a breast feeding woman that is >5 rem (0.05 Sv) TEDE or has resulted in unintended permanent functional damage to an organ or a physiological system of the child, as determined by a physician.

Notification consists of first telephoning the NRC Operations Center no later than the next calendar day after discovery of the event, followed by a written report to the appropriate NRC Regional Office within 15 days that includes: licensee's name; name of prescribing physician; brief description of event; why event occurred; effect, if any, on embryo/fetus or nursing child; actions taken, if any, to prevent recurrence; and certification that licensee notified pregnant individual or mother (or responsible relative or guardian), and if not, why not. The report must not contain any information that could lead to identification of the individual or child. The licensee must also provide an annotated copy of the report to the referring physician no later than 15 days after the discovery of the event, with the name of the pregnant individual or the nursing child and his or her Social Security or other identifying number.

A licensee must provide notification of the event to the referring physician and also notify the pregnant individual or mother (both hereafter referred to as the mother), no later than 24 hours after discovery of the event, unless the referring physician personally informs the licensee either that he or she will inform the mother or that, based on medical judgment, telling the mother would be harmful. The licensee is not required to notify the mother without first consulting with the referring physician. If the referring physician or mother cannot be reached within 24 hours, the licensee must make the appropriate notifications as soon as possible thereafter (if necessary, notification may be made to a responsible relative or guardian). The licensee may not delay any appropriate medical care for the embryo/fetus or for the nursing child. If a verbal notification is made, the licensee must inform the mother that a written description of the event can be obtained upon request.

16.7.2 Discussion of the Requirements

The required reports are self-explanatory. The reporting requirements under § 20.2201 appear to be overly conservative and ambiguous. For example, licensees must notify NRC immediately after discovery that 1 mCi (37 MBq) of ^{131}I is lost, stolen, or missing "under such circumstances that it appears to the licensee that an exposure could result to persons in unrestricted areas." The degree of exposure is not specified. Licensees must also notify NRC within 30 days if 10 μCi (370 kBq) of ^{131}I is lost, stolen, or missing.

16.7.3 Suggested Procedures for Compliance

Licensees should be able easily to develop forms for each of the required reports based on the information in this chapter. It is anticipated that the reporting of some of these events (e.g., medical events and unauthorized medical exposure of embryo/fetus) will be rare but could occur. Permanent functional damage to an organ (i.e., the thyroid) is also highly likely with Na ^{131}I. A functioning thyroid exists in an embryo/fetus at approximately 12 weeks gestation.

16.8 Safety Instruction for Workers and Personnel

16.8.1 Pertinent Regulations

10 CFR 20.1301 Dose limits for individual members of the public.

(a) (1) TEDE to individual members of the public must not exceed 0.1 rem (1 mSv) in a year.

(c) Licensees may apply for prior NRC authorization to operate up to an annual dose limit for an individual member of the public of 0.5 rem (5 mSv).

10 CFR 35.310 Safety instruction.

Licensees must provide radiation safety instruction (and retain a record of individuals receiving instruction), initially and at least annually, to personnel caring for patients or human research subjects who cannot be released under § 35.75. The instruction must be commensurate with the duties of the personnel and include:

(1) Patient or human research subject control;
(2) Visitor control, including:
  (a) Routine visitation to hospitalized individuals in accordance with § 20.1301(a)(1); and
  (b) Visitation authorized in accordance with § 20.1301(c).
(3) Contamination control;
(4) Waste control; and
(5) Notification of the RSO or his or her designee and the AU if the patient or the human research subject has a medical emergency or dies.

16.8.2 Discussion of the Requirements

For personnel involved in radiopharmaceutical therapy in instances in which a treated patient or human research subject cannot be released under § 35.75, safety instruction is required initially and at least annually. These personnel may be nuclear medicine or radiation oncology staff, referring physicians, or members of the nursing staff. This safety instruction should be commensurate with the duties of the personnel and include safe handling, patient control, visitor control, contamination control, waste control, and notification of the RSO and AU if the patient has a medical emergency or dies. Part 20 requirements allow licensees to permit visitors to a patient who cannot be released to receive a dose >0.1 rem (1 mSv), provided the dose does not exceed 0.5 rem (5 mSv) and the AU has determined before the visit that it is appropriate.

Licensees also might determine that housekeeping staff, although not likely to receive doses in excess of applicable public dose limits, should be (for example) informed of the nature of the licensed material and the meaning of the radiation symbol, instructed not to touch the licensed material, and told to remain out of the room. Providing minimal instruction to ancillary staff (e.g., housekeeping, security, etc.) may assist in controlling abnormal events.

16.8.3 Suggested Procedures for Compliance

Safety instruction for professional staff (e.g., AU, RSO, nuclear medicine technologist) in diagnostic nuclear medicine were discussed previously in this book. In addition to this instruction, licensees must also provide instruction, initially and at least annually, commensurate with the duties of the personnel, in:

(1) Patient or human research subject control;
(2) Visitor control;
(3) Contamination control;
(4) Waste control; and
(5) What to do in the event that a patient or human research subject has a medical emergency or dies.

As an example, instruction should include authorized visitation exceeding the 0.1 rem (1 mSv) public dose limit if:

(1) The visitor's radiation dose will not exceed 0.5 rem (5 mSv); and
(2) The authorized user has determined before the visit that it is appropriate (see section 16.5). It may be useful to develop a video or readable instructional materials to facilitate the training of new staff before they deal with a radionuclide therapy patient.

If staff and procedures have not changed in a given year, the instruction should be minimized. New employees must receive appropriate safety instruction, but there should be no requirement to continuously train those personnel who are already adequately trained. The requirement of annual instruction to veteran personnel seems overly burdensome. *Note:* Licensees may want to consider applying to the NRC for an exemption to this continual radiation safety instruction requirement as it applies to adequately trained, veteran employees caring for radionuclide therapy patients who are required to be confined to a hospital room.

16.9 Audit Program

16.9.1 Pertinent Regulations

10 CFR 20.1101 Radiation protection programs. Licensees must review, at least annually, the radiation protection program content and implementation.

10 CFR 20.2102 Records of radiation protection programs. Licensees must maintain records of audits and other reviews of the radiation protection program content and implementation.

10 CFR 35.26 Radiation protection program changes. Licensees may revise their radiation protection programs without NRC approval if certain conditions are met.

16.9.2 Discussion of the Requirements

Licensees must review and/or audit their radiation protection program content, implementation, and effectiveness on an annual basis (or more frequently, if deficiencies are identified). This is important so that any violations or radiation safety concerns that may be identified can be corrected in a timely manner. Not all deficiencies must result in corrective actions, as long as appropriate reasons can be given. These reviews may also indicate that certain procedures and/or requirements should be minimized or even eliminated. In this case, the licensee should appropriately alter their radiation protection policies and implementing procedures and/or apply to the NRC for an exemption from the applicable requirements in Parts 19, 20, 30, and 35 as discussed earlier in this book.

16.9.3 Suggested Procedures for Compliance

All aspects of the licensee's radiation protection program must be reviewed on an annual basis. If any deficiencies are identified sooner, the appropriate areas of the program should be reviewed at that time. The audit should be performed with the following three questions in mind:

(1) What can happen?
(2) How likely is it?
(3) What are the consequences?

Form 16.1 contains a list of the items to be checked and can be used for auditing the radiation protection program for radiopharmaceutical therapy licensees.

Note: An audit program for diagnostic nuclear medicine was detailed earlier in this volume. Additional requirements apply to radiopharmaceutical therapy, and only those are included in Form 16.1 for auditing the radiation protection program. Diagnostic nuclear medicine and radiopharmaceutical therapy licensees will need to combine Forms 9.1 and 16.1 for a comprehensive audit form.

FORM 16.1

Radiation Protection Program Audit for Radiopharmaceutical Therapy

Date of review: ______________________ Date of last review: ______________________

Reviewer: ______________________ Date: ______________
(Name and signature)

Management Review: ______________________ Date: ______________
(Name and signature)

Audit History

1. Were previous audits conducted annually (or sooner, if necessary)?
2. Were records of previous audits maintained?
3. Were any deficiencies identified during previous audits?
4. Were corrective actions taken?

Training and Experience

1. Does the authorized user (AU) meet Nuclear Regulatory Commission (NRC) training requirements?
2. Does the radiation safety officer (RSO) meet NRC training requirements?

   (Do the authorized nuclear pharmacist [ANP] and authorized medical physicist [AMP] meet NRC training requirements?)
3. Is the RSO fulfilling all duties?

   If the RSO was changed, was the license amended?
4. Recentness of training?

Occupational Dose Limits

1. Are dose limits for adults maintained?
2. Is internal dose monitored, if required?

Radiation Surveys

1. Are exposure rate surveys performed at the end of each day in all appropriate areas when unsealed byproduct material requiring a written directive was used?

Written Directives

1. Are written directive procedures in place?
2. Do written directives contain required information?
3. Are written directives signed and dated by AU before dosage administration?
4. Is patient's or human research subject's identity verified before each dosage administration?
5. Is each dosage administration verified to be in accordance with written directive?
6. Are proper written revisions made, if any, to existing written directives?
7. Are supervised individuals instructed in and required to follow written directive procedures?

Release of Individuals Containing Unsealed Byproduct Material

1. Is patient release correctly authorized?
2. Are appropriate instructions given to released patients?
3. Are appropriate instructions given to breast feeding women?

Safety Procedures for Treatment When Patients are Hospitalized

1. Are patient rooms adequate?
2. Are patient rooms posted with "Radioactive Materials" signs?
3. Is visitor control adequate?
4. Are materials and items removed from patients' rooms handled appropriately?
5. Are adequate surveys performed during period of confinement and before room release for unrestricted use?
6. Are proper procedures in place in the event of patient medical emergency or death?
7. If emergency or death occurred, were procedures followed?

Records/Reports

1. Are appropriate records kept?
2. Are appropriate reports written?

Safety Instruction for Workers and Personnel

1. Is adequate safety instruction being given to personnel caring for patients who cannot be released under § 35.75?
2. Is instruction being given at least annually?

Audit Findings

1. Summary of findings:
   a. Any appropriate program changes (any procedures identified that need to be corrected or any that could be minimized or eliminated?)
   b. Any exemptions from applicable requirements that should be requested?
2. Corrective and preventive actions:

17 License Application

17.1 Application Process and License Issuance

To apply for a Nuclear Regulatory Commission (NRC) license in diagnostic nuclear medicine and radiopharmaceutical therapy (utilizing unsealed sources for which a written directive is needed) an applicant must do the following (§ 35.12):

(1) File an original and one copy of NRC Form 313, Application for Material License, that includes the facility diagram, equipment, and training and experience qualifications of the radiation safety officer (RSO) and authorized user(s) (AU) (if applicable, also authorized medical physicists [AMPs] and authorized nuclear pharmacists [ANPs]); and

(2) Have management sign the application.

The submission of written procedures to meet the requirements of the applicable regulations is not required as part of the license application process. However, the applicant must provide a commitment to "develop, document, and implement" these procedures as they will be examined during NRC inspections. The suggested procedures detailed in Chapter 5 of this volume can be used for these purposes. The applicant also must provide any other information requested by the NRC in its review of the application. (For license amendments and/or renewals, the reader is referred to earlier sections of this volume and to § 35.12 and §35.13.)

The NRC will issue a license for the medical use of byproduct material if (§ 35.18):

(1) The applicant has filed NRC Form 313, *Application for Material License,* in accordance with the instructions in § 35.12;

(2) The applicant has paid any applicable fee as provided in 10 CFR Part 170;

(3) The Commission finds the applicant equipped and committed to observe the required safety standards established for the protection of the public health and safety; and

(4) The applicant meets the requirements of 10 CFR Part 30.

The first step in filing for an NRC materials license is to complete NRC Form 313. The form includes 13 items; items 1–4, 12, and 13 can be completed on the form itself, whereas items 5–11 require supplementary pages. The following section explains and provides suggested responses, item by item, for all the information requested on NRC Form 313 for licensed facilities seeking a specific license of limited scope to use unsealed byproduct material prepared for medical use for which a written directive is required (i.e., § 35.300 material). It will be assumed for purposes of this license application that applicants requesting use of § 35.300 materials will also be requesting use of § 35.100 and § 35.200 materials (described earlier in this volume).

17.1.1 Item 1. License Action Type

Check the box for a new license (for amendments or renewals, see material in the diagnostic section of this book).

17.1.2 Item 2. Applicant's Name and Mailing Address

The legal name of the applicant's facility must be given. This is the entity that has direct control over use of the radioactive material. Pertinent divisions or departments within hospitals may not be listed. The mailing address must also be provided.

Note: The NRC must be notified before control of the license is transferred, whenever bankruptcy proceedings are initiated, or when a licensee decides to permanently cease licensed activities:

(1) **Notification of Transfer of Control**
Licensees must provide full information and obtain NRC's written consent before transferring control of the license (§ 30.34(b)). A

simple name change that does not involve transfer of control of the license or mailing address change only requires written notification with NRC no later than 30 days after the date of the change.

(2) **Notification of Bankruptcy Proceedings** Immediately (i.e., within 24 hours) after the filing of a bankruptcy petition, a licensee must notify the NRC. This is because the NRC wants to ensure that there will be no public health and safety concerns. The licensee remains responsible for compliance with all regulatory requirements.

(3) **Termination of Activities/License Termination** For therapeutic radionuclide licenses, license termination does not require much effort, because the total inventory of licensed material will not exceed regulatory limits and because the half-lives of the unsealed byproduct materials used are so short. The NRC must be notified, in writing, within 60 days, when the license has expired or a decision has been made to permanently cease licensed activities at the entire site or in any separate building that contains residual radioactivity. Licensees must certify the disposition of licensed materials and, if appropriate, that the facility is not contaminated, to facilitate decommissioning (i.e., release of the site for unrestricted use). For the interested reader, Subpart E to 10 CFR Part 20 describes the radiological criteria for license termination.

17.1.3 Item 3. Address(es) Where Licensed Material will be Used

The address should specify a street address, not a post office box, because the address must be sufficient to allow NRC inspectors to find the facility location.

17.1.4 Item 4. Contact Person

A person knowledgeable about the application and the facility should be listed as the contact person (typically the proposed RSO), because the NRC will contact this individual if there are questions about the application. The telephone number of this individual must also be included.

17.1.5 Item 5. Radioactive Material

The form specifies:

a. Element and mass number;
b. Chemical and/or physical form; and
c. Maximum amount that will be possessed at any one time.

Because this is an application for a specific license of limited scope for the use of § 35.300 material as well as § 35.100 and § 35.200 materials, the applicant should provide the following information:

a. Any byproduct material included in 10 CFR 35.100, 10 CFR 35.200 and 10 CFR 35.300;
b. Any; and
c. "As needed" for § 35.100 and § 35.200 materials and "300 mCi" for § 35.300 materials.

Note: The 300 mCi are not required by regulations but suggested by guidance given in NUREG-1556, Volume 9. For licensees who will treat mainly hyperthyroid patients and an occasional thyroid cancer patient, 300 mCi may be adequate. For those licensees who plan to treat multiple thyroid cancer patients at the same time and/or who expect to use other ^{131}I-labeled agents, a possession limit of several curies is more appropriate.

17.1.6 Item 6. Purpose(s) for Use of Licensed Material

The applicant can define the purposes of use by providing the following statements:

(1) "Any uptake, dilution, and excretion procedure approved in 10 CFR 35.100";
(2) "Any imaging and localization procedure approved in 10 CFR 35.200"; and
(3) "Any use of unsealed byproduct material approved in 10 CFR 35.300."

17.1.7 Item 7. Individual(s) Responsible for Radiation Safety Program and Their Training and Experience

The NRC requires that an applicant be qualified by training and experience to use licensed materials for the purposes requested in such a manner as to protect health and minimize danger to life or property. For therapeutic radionuclide licensees, the personnel who typically have a role in the radiation protection program are the RSO and the AU physician(s). Their training and experience (see Chapter 15 for § 35.300 material and Chapter 8 for § 35.100 and § 35.200 materials) must be documented in the license application (if ANPs and/or AMPs are involved, their training and experience must also be provided). NRC Form 313A, Training and Experience and Preceptor Statement, may be used for this purpose.

(1) Radiation Safety Officer

Applicants must provide the name of the proposed RSO and credentials demonstrating adequate training and experience. In addition, the applicant should supply documentation indicating that management has delegated the authority for the day-to-day oversight of the radiation protection program to the RSO and that the RSO has agreed in writing to be responsible for implementing the radiation protection program.

(2) Authorized Users

Applicants must provide the name of the proposed AU(s) and credentials demonstrating adequate training and experience in the uses requested.

17.1.8 Item 8. Safety Instruction for Individuals Working in Restricted Areas

Individuals working in the vicinity of licensed material must have adequate safety instruction as described in sections 9.14 and 16.8. Licensees must have written policies and procedures in place. However, no response is necessary on the license application.

17.1.9 Item 9. Facilities and Equipment

The facilities and equipment must be adequate to protect health and minimize danger to life or property (§ 30.33(a)(2)). According to § 35.12, the application must include a diagram of the facility and describe the equipment necessary for the radiation protection program. Refer to Chapter 10 for information on the facility diagram, equipment, and necessary statements to be provided in the application. In addition, applicants should describe the room(s) in which patients will be housed if they cannot be released under 10 CFR 35.75. This discussion should include a description of shielding, if applicable.

17.1.10 Item 10. Radiation Protection Program

The radiation protection program was described in Chapters 9 and 16, along with suggested written radiation protection policies and implementing procedures to ensure compliance with all applicable NRC regulations. Applicants should provide a statement such as: "We have developed and will document and implement written procedures for a radiation protection program that will ensure compliance with all applicable NRC regulations and the security and safe use of unsealed byproduct material in diagnostic nuclear medicine and radiopharmaceutical therapy procedures. The program addresses training and experience requirements for the RSO and AU(s) (and ANP or AMP, if applicable) and each of the following:

(1) Occupational dose limits;
(2) Dose limits for members of the public;
(3) Minimization of contamination/spill procedures;
(4) Material receipt and accountability/ordering, receiving, and opening packages;
(5) Radiation surveys and calibration of survey instruments;
(6) Caution signs and posting requirements;
(7) Labeling containers, vials, and syringes;
(8) Determining patient dosages;
(9) Sealed source inventory and leak testing;
(10) Waste disposal and decay-in-storage;
(11) Records;
(12) Reports;
(13) Safety instruction for workers and personnel;
(14) Audit program;
(15) Mobile diagnostic nuclear medicine services (if applicable);
(16) Written directives;
(17) Release of individuals containing unsealed byproduct material; and
(18) Safety procedures for treatment when patients are hospitalized."

Note: The necessary radiation protection program elements for each of the 18 areas in the above list can be found in both the diagnostic and therapy sections of this book.

17.1.11 Item 11. Waste Management

Licensed materials must be disposed of in accordance with NRC requirements; these have been described in section 9.11 and additional suggested procedures are given in Chapter 16.5 for therapeutic applications. Applicants should provide a statement such as: "We have developed and will document and implement written waste disposal procedures in accordance with the applicable regulations."

17.1.12 Item 12. Fees

Enter the appropriate fee category from 10 CFR 170.31. For specific licenses of limited scope, this is category 7 for medical licenses, subcategory C. The fee amount must be enclosed with the application.

17.1.13 Item 13. Certification

Typically, a representative of the legal entity filing the application should sign and date the application. This individual must be authorized to make binding commitments and to sign official documents on behalf of the applicant. An application for licensing a medical facility must be signed by the applicant's management, because, as previously discussed, signing the application acknowledges management's commitment and responsibilities for the radiation protection program.

Note: It is a criminal offense to make a willful false statement or representation on this application or any other correspondence with the NRC (18 U.S.C. 1001).